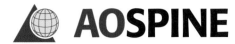

Michael J Lee | Daniel C Norvell | Joseph R Dettori | Andrea C Skelly | Jens R Chapman

SMART Approach to Spine Clinical Research

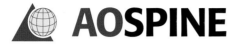

Michael J Lee | Daniel C Norvell | Joseph R Dettori | Andrea C Skelly | Jens R Chapman

SMART Approach to Spine Clinical Research

63 Figures and tables

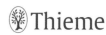

Design and layout: nougat GmbH, CH-4056 Basel
Illustrations: nougat GmbH, CH-4056 Basel
Production: AO Education Institute, CH-8600 Dübendorf

Library of Congress Cataloging-in-Publication Data is available from the publisher.

Copyright © 2013 by AOSpine, Switzerland, Clavadelerstrasse 8, CH-7270 Davos Platz
Distribution by Georg Thieme Verlag, Rüdigerstrasse 14, DE-70469 Stuttgart and
Thieme New York, 333 Seventh Avenue, New York, NY 10001, USA

ISBN: 9783131750617
E-ISBN: 9783131750716

Contributors

Editors

Michael J Lee, MD
Department of Orthopedics and Sports Medicine
Harborview Medical Center
University of Washington
1959 Pacific Street NE
Seattle, WA 98195
USA

Daniel C Norvell, PhD
Spectrum Research, Inc.
705 S 9th Street, Suite 203
Tacoma, WA 98405
USA

Joseph R Dettori, PhD, MPH
Spectrum Research, Inc.
705 S 9th Street, Suite 203
Tacoma, WA 98405
USA

Andrea C Skelly, PhD, MPH
Spectrum Research, Inc.
705 S 9th Street, Suite 203
Tacoma, WA 98405
USA

Jens R Chapman, MD
Department of Orthopedics and Sports Medicine
Harborview Medical Center
University of Washington
325 Ninth Avenue, Box 359798
Seattle, WA 98104-2499
USA

Authors

Paul A Anderson, MD
Professor Department of Orthopedics and Rehabilitation
University of Wisconsin
UWMF Centennial Bldg
1685 Highland Ave, 6th floor
Madison, WI 53705-2281
USA

Erika D Brodt, BSc
Spectrum Research, Inc.
705 S 9th Street, Suite 203
Tacoma, WA 98405
USA

Joseph S Cheng, MD
Department of Neurological Surgery
Vanderbilt University Medical Center
T-4224 Medical Center North
Nashville, TN 37232-2380
USA

Michael G Fehlings, MD, PhD
Department of Neurosurgery
University of Toronto
4 West, Room 449
399 Bathurst Street
Toronto, Ontario M5T 2S8
Canada

Nora B Henrickson, PhD, MPH
Spectrum Research, Inc.
705 S 9th Street, Suite 203
Tacoma, WA 98405
USA

Jeffrey T Hermsmeyer, BSc
Spectrum Research, Inc.
705 S 9th Street, Suite 203
Tacoma, WA 98405
USA

Preface

Despite decades of published clinical reports and studies, quality research is not common in the literature. Historically, much of the practice of medicine has been shaped by cumulative experiences, anecdotal evidence, and studies without control groups. While there is value in these reports and certainly they were the best evidence available at the time of publication, today there is a greater push to improve the quality of our studies and practice evidence-based medicine.

Most quality journals now require authors to provide a certain level of evidence for their studies. There are several systems using different descriptors for the level of evidence. In general, these systems focus mostly on study design and methods criteria to evaluate the potential for bias. These grades range from high (good-quality randomized controlled trials [RCTs]) to moderate (nonrandomized comparative studies), to low (case series and authors' opinions). The impact of evidence goes far beyond each individual study. Along with the mounting volume of published studies, we now have systems that grade an entire body of literature on a given topic. These systems take into account the full body of studies on a topic and render an overall strength of evidence. The Grades of Recommendation Assessment, Development and Evaluation (GRADE) system is the most common for providing a global assessment of evidence, which in turn facilitates the application of a "strong" or "weak" recommendation "for" or "against" a treatment or procedure. The grading of the overall body of evidence on a specific intervention not only influences medical practice, but also increasingly influences payer policies on reimbursement for various procedures. Hence, it behooves practicing spine surgeons to design and participate in clinical studies that produce the highest quality of evidence if we want to have an impact on future healthcare decisions and delivery.

Systematic reviews, which have recently become more frequent and popular, clearly highlight the shortage of quality evidence available in the literature. Consider any systematic review and note the substantial contrast between initial numbers of citations examined to the final number of studies included in the review, especially in comparative effectiveness reviews where only studies including a comparison or control group are included.

Importantly, however, high-quality studies do not necessarily have to be double-blind RCTs. There is no level I evidence proving that jumping out of an airplane with a parachute results in significantly less injury and death than jumping without a parachute. Yet, it is not advisable to test this hypothesis. In many cases, such as in trauma, it is extremely challenging to perform a randomized trial because of the unpredictability of the injury and the heterogeneity of the sample population. It is also often difficult to blind the assessment of outcomes to the treatment rendered. Thus, often what is observed in the literature, while methodologically not the highest quality possible, does represent the best evidence that is available. However, by understanding the precepts and design characteristics that go into proper study planning, you should always try to design a study with the highest possible level of evidence.

Frequently, new techniques are introduced into the literature as a case series soon to be followed by retrospective comparative studies, then prospective comparative trials. All of these studies are of value at the time, as a reasonable progression of understanding the safety and effectiveness of a new treatment. However, if one were to publish a case series on his or her cases of lumbar laminectomy for the treatment of lumbar spinal stenosis, such a low-quality design on a banal subject would likely contribute little to the literature discussion regarding the comparative safety or effectiveness of this surgical technique. This is something to keep in mind when balancing your time, funding, and professional development.

The purpose of this book is to assist you in planning a quality scientific study, regardless of your research experience. Quality scientific studies can range from simple question/answer, small clinical studies to complex analyses of double-blind RCTs. Planning is only one phase of a clinical study but arguably the most important. Without a well-thought out plan, a perfectly executed study will yield compromised results. The phases of study operations and reporting are not addressed in any detail unless it overlaps with an important planning concept. For example, this book does not teach the reader how to perform complex statistical analyses or complicated multi-site trials. However, this book does provide you with elements of these concepts as they relate to study planning. In many chapters, common methodological flaws and misconceptions are addressed.

There are many interrelated components that must be considered when embarking on a research project. As with any journey, a plan that outlines the various processes, modes of transportation, and milestones is needed. The precepts laid out in this book provide you with the elements to help you plan your research journey. We call it the SMART-B approach, which stands for:

- **Study question**
- **Searching the literature**
- **Study design**
- **Measurements**
- **Analysis**
- **Resources**
- **Timing**
- **Bias reduction**

While this is not a cookbook on how to write a study protocol, the SMART-B concepts provide the appropriate framework for creating a quality study protocol. The SMART-B concepts will facilitate your success and assist you in making a high-quality contribution to the body of evidence in your field. They will promote a greater appreciation for the aspects of a study that make or break it in terms of credibility, thus enhancing your critical appraisal skills.

You will note that following the SMART-B approach positions your research nicely for the publication process. Chapter 9: Special topics also assists you with honing your critical appraisal skills. Even if you never publish your study, you will need to be able to critically evaluate the literature in order to make the best treatment decisions for your patients. Special topics related to exploring which patients may benefit the most or the least from procedures, information on registries and their use, and the use of evidence in policy formulation provide you with insight on additional applications of the SMART-B approach for the creation and use of evidence. These sections provide food for thought for all researchers on some of the next steps in applying these concepts and the ramifications of producing or not producing high-quality studies.

We have attempted to weave in several case examples throughout the chapters to make the book practical and user-friendly. We hope that this will be an important resource for all spine surgeons interested in planning, executing, and evaluating research.

Enjoy your journey!

Jens R Chapman
Michael J Lee
Daniel C Norvell

Foreword/Acknowledgments

"Doctors have been exposed—you always will be exposed—to the attacks of those persons who consider their own undisciplined emotions more important than the world's most bitter agonies—the people who would limit and cripple and hamper research because they fear research may be accompanied by a little pain and suffering."

– Joseph Rudyard Kipling

Although physicians have spent decades learning, training, and practicing medicine, the large majority of physicians do not formally perform research. Yet in our practices and in our own minds, we are constantly seeking to improve the care of our patients. We are constantly observing treatments and characterizing patients and outcomes. "Since the last few patients did not do so well when I did the surgery this way, I am going to change how I do this." "What happens if I sprinkle Vancomycin powder in the wound before I close?" Although our practice preferences may be more testimonial than true scientific research, clearly they are motivated by the same spirit of asking a question and seeking the answer. We are all striving to improve the care we deliver to patients and advance our knowledge.

In the past a scientific exchange of ideas may have been sufficient enough to effect change in practice. However, in this ever-evolving healthcare world, practice oversight is expanding. Medical decisions are increasingly being influenced by nonclinicians and bureaucrats. The denial of healthcare procedures is being justified by third-party payers citing a lack of scientific evidence. Thus, the advancement of medical knowledge and practice through structured research is of paramount importance.

Indeed, the notion of research for many physicians is associated with more than just a little "pain and suffering". For many physicians, the idea of performing research rarely goes beyond a residency or fellowship requirement. They may want to contribute to the literature, but are discouraged by the onerous process. The purpose of this book is to ease some of that "pain and suffering" in conducting scientific research. We believe that this book will allow readers to envision a pathway to contributing to the literature and facilitate that process.

A book such as this would not be possible without the commitment and efforts of many individuals. Specifically, we are indebted to the authors and colleagues at Spectrum Research, Inc. who have devoted their time and effort to this work. We are particularly grateful to AOSpine, AO Education Institute under the leadership of Urs Rüetschi, and Carl Lau. We would like to thank Vidula Bhoyroo, Michael Gleeson, and Thea Swanson for proofreading our manuscript. Our thanks also go to Sandro Isler at nougat GmbH for the wonderful book design and illustrations. And most importantly, we would like to thank our loved ones for affording us the time on weekends and evenings to work on this important book.

Michael J Lee
Daniel C Norvell
Joseph R Dettori
Andrea C Skelly
Jens R Chapman

Table of Contents

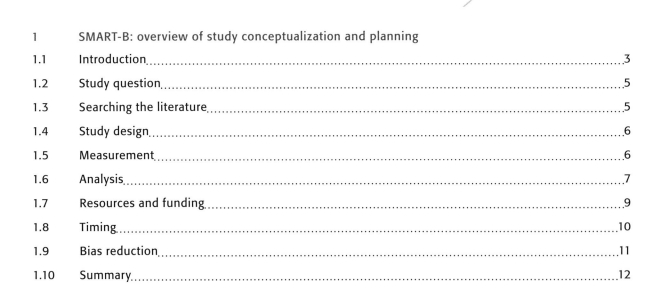

A goal without a plan is just a wish.
SMART-B: your road map to a successful study.
Chapters and milestones.

1   SMART-B: overview of study conceptualization and planning

1.1   Introduction

A journey of any significant complexity requires planning and a map for you to arrive at your destination efficiently, safely, and successfully.

☞ **Without sufficient preparation, organization, and an efficient, cost-effective route for getting you to your destination, you may get lost and/or possibly stuck at a milepost you did not want to visit.**

By not _following the map_, that short cut you thought you remembered may lead to a dead end or detours, which might significantly extend your journey. In clinical research, we call this map the study protocol. The SMART-B approach to planning should assist you in writing your study protocol.

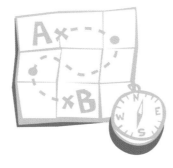

The purpose of this chapter is to provide an overview of the basic stepping stones that comprise the SMART-B approach for planning clinical research. Each of the subsequent chapters provides more detail about the various topics. Throughout the book, you will be exposed to real-world case examples to which the SMART-B approach will be applied to assist you with understanding the components and adapting them to your research question. Here we set the stage for the primary components:

S tudy question	(chapter 2)
S earching the literature	(chapter 3)
S tudy design	(chapter 4)
M easurements	(chapter 5)
A nalysis	(chapter 6)
R esources	(chapter 7)
T iming	(chapter 7)
B ias reduction	(chapter 8)

Performing quality research is a complicated journey. The goal is to have a well-reported research study from which colleagues, healthcare providers, researchers, and policymakers can draw reasonable inferences that are valid from a methodological perspective and clinically useful. It is unfortunate that a large percentage of research in the medical literature is of poor quality and contains a number of avoidable errors. In this era of evidence-based medicine and the linking of reimbursement decisions to the quality of evidence available, it is important that new as well as more seasoned researchers seek ways of enhancing study quality. This in turn potentially enhances the quality of evidence available overall.

☞ Thus, it is becoming increasingly important that new study reports meet a higher standard and be able to withstand scrutiny by those beyond the immediate professional group.

The purpose of this book is to provide a map for planning and organizing a research project in a way that reduces errors and bias (random and systematic) so that valid inferences can be drawn. Many of the planning concepts overlap or influence the execution of a study. However, this book does not cover the details of study execution. It provides you with a map to making a meaningful contribution toward improving the quality of evidence available on a given topic, regardless of the study design you choose.

Planning a successful study requires consideration of various interrelated factors. In order to effectively perform and analyze the study, a systematic approach is needed. In order to create a high-quality report of study findings (and publish them), documentation of the process as well as the findings are required. The SMART-B approach facilitates understanding of these factors and processes to assist you with planning and reporting quality research. Performing your own research using these principles will also enhance your critical thinking skills on what to consider when appraising published research in your field.

What does _SMART-B_ stand for and how can it help you with your project? The following is a quick overview. Each of the SMART-B components is fully discussed in subsequent chapters.

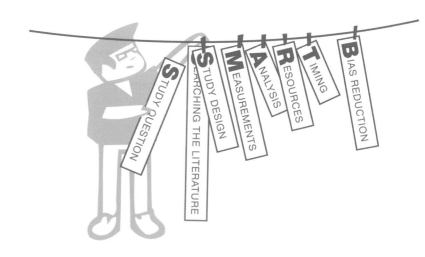

1.2 Study question

Formulating a clear, answerable study question(s) is the single most important step in research. Everything that is planned, executed, analyzed, and reported must link back to the study question. The study question is the foundation for all the next steps in planning and executing a study. It is the basis of your game plan.

A well-specified study question provides information about the patients to be studied, treatments to be compared (or factors that need to be studied), and primary outcomes that are important. Using the patients, intervention, comparison, and outcomes (PICO) algorithm for treatment (and many diagnostic studies) provides a structure for stipulating who and what is to be studied, what interventions are to be compared, and which outcomes are most meaningful. Similarly, the patients, prognostic factors, and outcomes (PPO) algorithm for prognostic studies allows you to specify which primary factors may influence risk for specific outcomes as well as potentially confounding factors. These algorithms assist you in organizing your thoughts and provide a basis for your inclusion and exclusion criteria.

1.3 Searching the literature

The study question (and PICO or PPO tables) in turn provides the framework for conducting a search of the literature on the topic. The search provides important insights into the appropriate study design. A reasonably thorough literature search is required for understanding what other research has been reported on the topic, what gaps there are in the evidence that your research might be able to fill, and what study design(s) may be most appropriate for answering your study question.

For example, if there have been a number of randomized controlled trials (RCTs) published on your study question, a formal systematic review with or without meta-analysis may be the most appropriate study design to answer your question.

On the other hand, if there are multiple case series published on a topic, doing an additional case series may not provide a meaningful addition to the quality of the evidence and does not advance the knowledge or the value of a given treatment to the extent that a methodologically rigorous comparative study would. If your question involves a rare disease or outcome and little is published on the topic, a well-designed case-control study may be the best option.

1.4   Study design

☞ **The strongest study design is the one which addresses your study question with the least opportunity for bias and provides for direct comparison of appropriate groups of participants when studying issues of efficacy, effectiveness, and safety.**

Although RCTs potentially have the least potential for bias, they cannot answer all questions, particularly related to safety and long-term outcomes. Thus, methodologically rigorous comparative observational studies may be the best design for some questions. Case series can provide some information and can be helpful for hypothesis generation. However, since they do not directly compare groups, they are of limited value in establishing effectiveness and safety. Chapter 4: Importance and implications of study design selection provides more detailed information on various study designs. Factors such as time and resources also need to be considered when designing your study and are discussed in chapter 7: Resources and timing.

Again, the most important first step is having a focused, answerable study question. "It doesn't matter how you get there if you don't know where you are going." This quote from a performance by the Flying Karamazov Brothers states the obvious about research.

☞ **Without solid, answerable study questions delineating where you want to go with your research, the path to getting there cannot be defined and will not be efficient.**

1.5   Measurement

Your study question, search of the literature, and study design inform what measurements you will need to make. What needs to be measured is whom, how, when, and why. When it comes to measurements, researchers often focus on outcomes. However, there are at least four categories of measurement:

- Baseline factors
- Treatment factors
- Perioperative and immediate posttreatment events
- Outcomes

Patient characteristics are an often under-reported or misreported set of measurements, but are extremely important to quantify and report. They potentially influence both the internal and external validity of your study. Diagnostic features, comorbidities, perioperative events, and any factors that might affect patient outcome need to be measured and reported for each study group. All these characteristics, features, and factors may be potential confounders of the relationship between your exposure of interest (eg, a surgical treatment) and the outcome (eg, patient function or adverse event). Planning for and measurement of these factors goes a long way toward evaluating the role of confounding, which is an important potential source of study bias.

1.6 Analysis

Your study question and PICO/PPO table provide you with a conceptualization of what is to be measured with respect to outcome. Now you need to specify what precise measurements or instruments are to be used. This is called operationalizing your measurements. For example, if your primary outcome of interest is patient function, how exactly will you measure and report it? Is a clinician-based measurement or a patient-reported measurement most appropriate? What is your goal in measuring it? Is there a measurement that directly quantifies the functional aspect that is important to your study? Will you use a validated functional measurement, such as the Oswestry Disability Index? What is your rationale for using the measurement? What are the strengths and limitations of the measurement for evaluating the truth about your outcome? What constitutes a clinically meaningful threshold for improvement in the measurement and how will you determine this?

What you want to measure and the method of measurement also form the basis of how you will calculate sample size (which is related to study power) and the fundamental types of statistical analysis that will be needed to evaluate the role of chance in your study.

Considerations regarding analysis must be addressed long before you collect your data and encompass more than testing for statistical significance. This is a complex topic, but if you have a SMART plan for your analysis and take time to understand some of the basic concepts of hypothesis testing using statistical methods, it is manageable and even fun! Again, the concepts outlined here are covered in more detail in subsequent chapters.

The analysis plan must be determined up front to ensure that the sample size is appropriate and that the proper data are abstracted or collected. It must directly flow from your study question, study design, primary outcome(s) of interest, and methods for measurement. Together with the study design, the type of data for your primary outcome (eg, dichotomous data such as yes or no, continuous data like a Visual Analog Scale score for pain) form the basis for sample size determination as well as the statistical tests of your hypothesis. Your plan needs to consider how you will analyze potential confounding factors and whether you are looking for differential benefit or harm in subpopulations (this will influence the sample size needed). A significant portion of the methods section of your paper will flow directly from your analysis plan. The internal

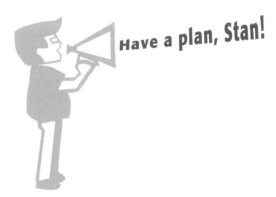

Have a plan, Stan!

validity of your study directly relates to your analysis plan and its tie-in to your study question as well as methods of recruiting and evaluating participants.

☞ **An analysis plan, carefully set out beforehand, minimizes any loss in time, resources, and opportunities in the end. It ensures that objectives are met and that appropriate hypotheses are being tested using the appropriate statistical methods. It is also a major contributor to the credibility of your research.**

In your analysis plan you will outline what types of statistical tests are appropriate to test your hypothesis and measure your objectives based on the study design and how your exposures and outcomes are measured. These are analytical statistics. Chapter 6: Analysis will empower you with some of the basic concepts related to evaluating associations and correlations. The general anatomy of test statistics and their roles in hypothesis testing are explained. Statistical testing is a means by which the role of chance is evaluated as an explanation for the observed results. A word of caution: one never "proves" something with statistical testing. It does, however, help us assess the likelihood that the effect we observed was or was not due to chance.

☞ **Analytical statistics cannot make up for poor study design or bias in the study, and statistical significance can be an artifact of study bias. A statistically significant finding may or may not be clinically significant.**

The correct interpretation of the results of statistical testing is as important as applying the correct statistical methods. This goes beyond looking at the P value! The P value only assesses the extent to which an observed affect may be due to chance. It needs to be put into context and a number of factors must be considered for meaningful interpretation of the results:

- Could the result be due to or influenced by bias in the study? What types of bias might be operating and how might this influence the result?
- What is the effect size and is it clinically meaningful (whether or not it is statistically significant)?
- How much variability is there in the estimate of effect size and how does this potentially influence the stability (and credibility) of the estimate?
- What does a statistically significant result for this study really mean?
- What are the limitations of the measurements or statistical approaches used?

These questions are also important to consider when doing critical appraisal of the literature. Having a basic understanding of these concepts will not only facilitate planning your own research, but also provide you with additional tools to put the research of others in context.

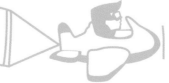

Statistics, testing, and interpretation: P values are not enough!

1.7   Resources and funding

Your study design and analysis plan need to take into consideration the resources (human and monetary) that are needed in order to execute, analyze, and report your study. There is always a need to balance what you would like to do with your research with the resources that are available, even if you have a multicenter RCT with funding from the National Institutes of Health in the United States!

Obviously, there is a need to consider whether you have access to funding for your study and what amount is available. Studies can be done with little or no external funding, if one is willing to put in the "sweat equity" to get it done and has access to a team that is willing to provide in-kind assistance in exchange for authorship.

Your resource requirements will be at least partly based on some basic questions:

☑ Do you need methodological assistance for study design and creating an analysis plan?

☑ Where and how will you get your data? Are data to be collected directly from patients or is abstraction of data needed or both? How much of this are you able/willing to do and how much needs to be done by someone else? Do you have a registry or database available, medical records, or can you afford the time and cost of a prospective study? Who owns the data and how accessible is it?

☑ How long will it take to collect the data (eg, for a 5-year prospective study, resources for all 5 years will be needed)?

☑ How will data be collected, checked, analyzed, interpreted, and reported? What expertise is needed for each component?

☑ What is needed with respect to computers (access to computers for data entry, programs, etc), Internet capability (eg, electronic data capture), and office supplies and processes (eg, copying/printing, telephone, fax, collating information)?

☑ How will the research get reported? What clinical or analytical expertise is needed to ensure the credibility of the report? Is assistance needed for figures, formatting, and similar tasks?

You must carefully think through the various tasks that need to be done related to study design, execution, analysis, and reporting. What expertise is needed to do which tasks and what "price", monetary or otherwise, will there be for each task? How much are you able and willing to do yourself? When might it be best to spend some money for assistance to ensure best use of your time and expertise and to ensure the highest possible quality for your study?

Building a good team is essential to the success of any project. A crucial piece that sometimes gets relegated to the sidelines is a realistic appraisal of the strengths and limitations of potential team members and possible collaborators. Who will be needed to get you where you need to go based on your strengths and limitations? What type of assistance will they provide? Who will specifically do what tasks and how will you keep them on track and motivated? Your team could include person(s) abstracting data and/or entering it into a computer, database experts, trained interviewers, study coordinators, methodologists, clinical experts in areas outside of your expertise, colleagues in your field, data analysts, and scientific writers. You may wear many of these hats, depending on your expertise, time, and resources. However, in general, it is difficult to implement any type of research project, particularly a high-quality project, without some involvement of others. Your choice of team members should be strategic and well-thought out.

1.8   Timing

Timing is another of the practical considerations that must be part of planning and executing your study. There are several components of time to consider:

- Timeline: How much time is needed from study concept to publication given your resources or professional demands? Factors that need to be considered here include:

  - Is a prospective or retrospective study most logical? What is realistic given your potential for resources? If prospective, how much time will it take for the various outcomes to manifest?
  - How long will the various tasks (eg, data collection, analysis, writing of the manuscript) take?
  - What are logical milestones that need to be accomplished to meet your timeline?
  - How much of your time is available to oversee, participate, and keep things on track?

- Timing of follow-up: Which measures should be performed at what time intervals (and why)? How long should follow-up be to allow effective evaluation of outcome(s)?

- Timeliness: How quickly should it be published? In other words, how time-sensitive is it? Does it need to be finished within a certain time frame?

1.9   Bias reduction

Bias is ubiquitous! As stated previously, the quality of much of the medical literature is poor, frequently due to biases and errors that could have been avoided with proper planning and implementation. Even RCTs have the potential for bias. Bias can significantly be reduced in nonrandomized studies without great expense. It comes down to planning.

☞ **Before you implement your study or analyze your data, it is very important that you implement methods to decrease or account for the influence of bias in your study design and analysis plan.**

A plan to reduce bias assists you in assuring that your study is credible versus incredible! While some criteria apply only to RCTs, most apply to any study design you choose. Primary potential sources of bias include:

- Patient selection
- Allocation of treatment
- Blind or independent assessment for important outcomes
- Use of reliable data and defined outcomes
- Applying co-interventions to each group equally
- Patient follow-up rate
- Adequate sample size
- Applying co-interventions to each group equally
- Validity of randomization process, concealment of treatment allocation and intention to treat (applies to RCTs)

These are some of the primary factors that form the basis of formal critical appraisal. The extent to which you are able to reduce these common sources of bias influences the internal validity (ie, the credibility) of your study particularly to those outside of professional circles who evaluate the quality of evidence.

Chapter 8: Bias reduction serves as an important check and balance for your study design, methods, and analysis plan. In some respects, it is one of the most important chapters in this book as it ties together many concepts described in previous chapters to help you finalize your overall study plan and execution. Do not skip this chapter!

1.10 Summary

- There are many interrelated components that must be considered when embarking on a research project. As with any journey, a plan that outlines the various processes, modes of transportation, and milestones is needed.

- Implementing the SMART-B concepts as your map to creating a quality study protocol for the planning of a high-quality study will facilitate your success and assist you in making an impactful contribution to the body of evidence in your field. It promotes a greater appreciation for the aspects that make or break a study in terms of credibility, thus enhancing your critical appraisal skills.

- In addition to detailed chapters on the topics above, chapter 9: Special topics gives you insights into specialized aspects of research, implications of research, and how it may be used in public policy.

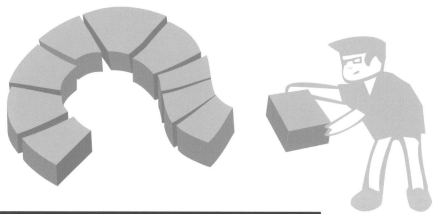

Are you asking the right question?
PICO and PPO, a systematic approach to creating a clinical question.

2　　Constructing a SMART study question

2.1　Introduction

Formulating a clear, focused, answerable study question(s) is the single most important step in research. Everything that is planned, executed, analyzed, and reported must link back to the study question(s) and related study objective(s). In this chapter, we focus on two steps for specifying a study question about a treatment comparison that will create the springboard for your study.

2.2   Initial refinement of your study question

Let us start with a case example. Below is the initial concept for the study we want to design:

Topic: Posterolateral instrumented fusion (PLF) versus interlaminar lumbar instrumented fusion (ILIF), a comparison of perioperative complications, fusion rates, and clinical outcomes.

Study objective: Determine if there is a difference between complication rates, fusion rates, and outcomes between two different arthrodesis techniques: ILIF and PLF.

Hypotheses:
• Fusion rates with PLF are significantly higher than fusion rates with ILIF
• Perioperative complication rates with PLF are also significantly higher than ILIF
• Improvements with clinical outcome will be significantly greater in the PLF group compared to the ILIF group

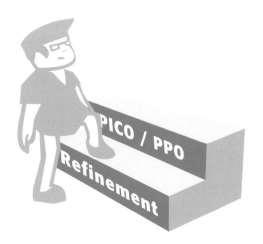

Desired claims at the end of the study: State whether or not there is a difference in the perioperative complication rates, fusion rates, and outcomes between PLF and ILIF.

At first glance it may seem that this is a specific, focused study question. If we consider what we have more carefully, however, we see that there are a number of questions that arise:

• What types of patients and pathology are to be studied and which should be excluded?
• An intervention (ILIF) and a comparator (PLF) are specified, but are there variations of these procedures or situations that we do not want to have in the study?
• What specific complications and outcomes are most important to measure and evaluate? What specific improvements need to be considered?
• Is it realistic or feasible to evaluate all hypotheses in a single study? Or should each be a separate study question?
• What is already published on this topic? Where are the gaps in the evidence and understanding that this study will address?
• What type of study is best suited to evaluate this topic and how will it add to the existing evidence on the topic?

This outline gives us the initial concept for the study. However, before it can be planned and executed, much further definition is needed.

☞ **Arriving at a concise, focused, and answerable study question is an iterative process. This requires answering specific questions and defining parameters that will be important to planning, executing, analyzing, and reporting your study.**

2.3   Conceptualizing your study in terms of PICO or PPO

Here is an example of refining the general study question. Suppose you are interested in the use of PLF and ILIF for treating spinal stenosis. **Table 2-1** is one logical progression for narrowing the focus of the study question.

Too broad	Somewhat more answerable	Improved focus
What is the comparative effectiveness and safety following PLF versus ILIF?	What is the comparative effectiveness and safety following PLF versus ILIF in the lumbar spine?	What is the comparative effectiveness and safety following PLF versus ILIF for spinal stenosis (with no greater than grade I spondylolisthesis) in the lumbar spine? or even … What is the comparative efficacy, effectiveness, and safety following single-level PLF versus single-level ILIF for spinal stenosis (with no greater than grade I spondylolisthesis) in the lumbar spine in symptomatic adult patients?

Table 2-1   Refining the study question from too broad to improved focus.

We have started to refine the question by specifying the condition or disease (spinal stenosis), aspects of the procedures (single level), and the patient population (symptomatic adults). There are still many unanswered questions and further specification is needed to create a laser-focused question. Are all patients with spinal stenosis to be included or should some be excluded? What specific safety factors, adverse events, or complications are important? What specific outcomes allow for comparative effectiveness or efficacy? Are you interested in efficacy or effectiveness? Efficacy refers to whether a drug or treatment works under ideal conditions. Randomized controlled trials provide the best evidence for efficacy as patients are carefully selected, specific protocols for treatment and assessment are followed, and generally biases are minimized. Even if a drug or treatment is efficacious, it may not work in a broader, unselected population. Effectiveness refers to whether a drug or treatment works in usual clinical practice in a broad range of patients, ie, in the real world. Observational studies are usually used to provide evidence of effectiveness.

For comparing treatments or designing diagnostic studies, specifying four main categories of basic study components can facilitate the creation of a laser-focused study question. A simple way to start framing an even more focused study question is to use the Patients, Intervention, Comparison, and Outcomes (PICO) approach. Taking time to complete a PICO table is important for framing your literature search and outlining your study conceptually.

The PICO table assists you in considering what specifically should be included, what should be excluded, what will be measured and in whom.

The PICO approach can be applied to treatment and diagnostic validation studies. For studies evaluating factors that influence outcomes (eg, risk factors for a poor outcome), the Patients, Prognostic factors, and Outcomes (PPO) approach is used (**Table 2-2**).

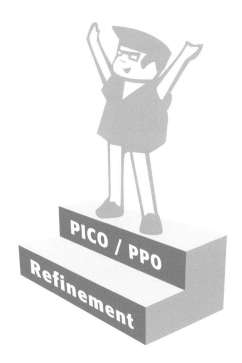

| | PICO | | PPO |
	PICO	Therapeutic	Diagnostic	Prognostic
Patients	What patient group?	What patient group?	**Patients**	What patient group?
Intervention	In what surgical treatment, procedure or implants are you interested?	What diagnostic procedure?	**Prognostic factors**	What primary prognostic (risk) factor might influence the outcomes?
Comparison	What is the comparison treatment?	Is there a gold standard or suitable reference standard?		What other factors might influence the outcomes?
Outcomes	In what outcomes are you interested (eg, pain)?	Are you interested in validity (eg, sensitivity/ specificity) and/ or reliability (eg, inter/intrarater reproducibility)?	**Outcomes**	In what outcomes are you interested (eg, nonunion)?

Table 2-2   Overview of PICO and PPO approaches.

PICO for treatment studies

Let's look at each component of PICO with a focus on its application to a study comparing two treatments.

Patients

Ideally, you want a homogeneous patient population. It is important to define the patient population in terms of all factors related to the condition of interest, patient demographic features (eg, age, gender), behaviors (eg, smoking), medical history, medications (eg, steroids, NSAIDS) that may influence outcomes, general health factors, comorbidities, factors that may be associated with the treatment selection (eg, location/severity of condition), and other factors that may be relevant to treatment selection or which may influence outcomes. Are patients with previous surgical interventions to be included or excluded? Are specific pathologies to be excluded?

Intervention

This may be a newer or novel treatment that is to be compared to a more standard treatment (called the comparator). In the example, ILIF will be the intervention of interest. Any variations of the procedures or technical aspects (approach, number of levels, use of specific devices, grafting procedures, etc) need to be specified as being included or excluded.

Comparison

This is the alternative, standard treatment to which the intervention is compared. This is your control group, which all comparative studies will have. Sometimes your question may not have a control group, such as when you are interested in safety, risks, or handling characteristics of a new implant or procedure. Posterolateral instrumented fusion is the comparator in the example provided. Again, are there variations of PLF or technical aspects that should be excluded?

Outcomes

Here you must decide what outcomes are important to your question. It is good to be specific and aim for the most important outcomes. Conceptual examples include patient reported outcomes, such as pain, function, and quality-of-life, as well as more clinical outcomes including nonunion, major complications, repeated surgery, or death. Chapter 5: Measurements describes factors to consider when choosing outcomes and methods of measurement.

	Inclusion	**Exclusion**
Patients	• Symptomatic adult patients with spinal stenosis • No greater than grade I spondylolisthesis • Evidence of spinal stenosis or claudication of the lumbar spine • No response to at least 6 months of conservative treatment	• Patients less than 18 years of age • Patients with spondylolistheis greater than grade I, isthmic spondylolisthesis, or other similar deformities • Thoracic or cervical spinal lesions • Patients with infection, tumor, neuromuscular disease, or autoimmune diseases • Patients with prior lumbar surgery at or adjacent to the index level • Patients with long-term steroid use
Intervention	• Instrumented ILIF • Direct lumbar decompression	• Non-instrumented ILIF
Comparison	• Instrumented PLF • Concurrent lumbar decompression	• Non-instrumented PLF • Interbody fusion

Outcomes	• Perioperative factors and complications
	  – Operative blood loss
	  – Infection
	• Fusion rates (fusion by 6 months)
	  – Clinical outcomes
	  – Function: Oswestry Disability Index (ODI)
	  – Pain: Visual Analog Scale (100-point scale)
	  – Return to normal activity
	  – Need for subsequent intervention
		• Costs, cost-effectiveness measures

Table 2-3   PICO table: What is the comparative effectiveness and safety following single-level PLF versus single-level ILIF for spinal stenosis of the lumbar spine?

If we apply the PICO approach to our conceptual study question, we see how we can begin to specify aspects of our study to inform more precisely what the study will involve (**Table 2-3**).

Specifying various parameters in the PICO table can then lead to further refinement of your study question and objectives.

Old question: Is there a difference in complication rates, fusion rates, and outcomes between two different arthrodesis techniques: ILIF and PLF?

Refined question reflecting PICO: In symptomatic adult patients with lumbar spinal stenosis (and no greater than grade I spondylolisthesis), are perioperative complications (eg, excessive blood loss), fusion rates, pain, and disability different in those who receive single-level PLF compared with those who receive single-level ILIF?

PICO for diagnostic studies

The PICO approach can also be applied to studies evaluating the validity (accuracy) and reliability of diagnostic studies. The following is a brief overview of some nuances for applying the PICO approach to diagnostic studies.

Patients

The study population must be composed of those with a broad spectrum of suspected disease and who are likely to have the test now or in the future. A broad spectrum would include patients with mild as well as more severe conditions, those presenting early as well as late, and those whose differential diagnosis may be commonly confused with the condition of interest. Thus, all factors that would describe the patient demographic and clinical features related to this spectrum should be specified. This is necessary whether you are doing a validation or a reliability study.

Intervention

This is the diagnostic test that you are seeking to validate. Specifics regarding the technical aspects (eg, equipment, planes of section, measurement protocols) and diagnostic criteria for determining a case and/or severity of a condition are needed.

Comparison

This is your referent or gold standard test. As with the test you are seeking to validate, the technical aspects and diagnostic criteria need to be delineated. Ideal reference standards are termed gold standards and in theory, provide the truth about the presence or absence of a condition or disease. They rarely exist, so the best reference or one that can be practically applied may be what is available and likely to accurately categorize patients according to disease status.

Outcomes

For validation studies, calculation of characteristics such as sensitivity, specificity, and predictive values are generally the outcomes of interest. The design of your study dictates whether all these are appropriate to calculate. For reliability studies, interclass correlation coefficients (ICC) or weighted Kappa coefficients generally provide the best outcomes measurements to consider.

PPO and prognostic studies

Perhaps you are interested in identifying factors that may be associated with a poor outcome. For example, suppose there is concern that patients with lumbar spinal stenosis who smoke are more likely to experience nonunion than those treated with other methods. Your study would then focus on evaluating if this is a risk factor for nonunion. This is the realm of a prognostic study.

Patients

As previously described, you want to specify the characteristics of patients that should be included and excluded. Patients who have the outcome of interest and those that do not have the outcome of interest should be included.

Prognostic factors

Prognostic factors or risk factors for the outcome of interest can be categorized in two broad groups:

- The primary factor(s) that you believe may be associated with the outcome
- Other factors that may potentially influence the relationship between the primary factor of interest and the outcome

Patients who have the prognostic factor of interest and those that do not should be included and compared.

Outcomes

The outcome of interest may be a positive outcome (eg, greater function) or poor outcome (eg, an adverse event).

The PPO table here would be helpful in answering the following clinical question (**Table 2-4**): In symptomatic patients with lumbar spinal stenosis, is one type of arthrodesis (ILIF or PLF) associated with nonunion after accounting for other factors (eg, smoking, NSAID use)?

	Inclusion	**Exclusion**
Patient	• Symptomatic adult patients • Spinal stenosis • No greater than grade I spondylolisthesis • No response to at least 6 months of conservative treatment	• Patients less than 18 years of age • Patients with spondylolisthesis greater than grade I, isthmic spondylolisthesis, or other similar deformities • Thoracic or cervical spine lesions • Patients with infection, tumor, neuromuscular disease, or autoimmune diseases • Patients with prior lumbar surgery at or adjacent to the index level • Patients with long-term steroid use
Prognostic factors	Primary factor of interest: • Procedure type (ILIF, PLF) Potential confounding factors: • Age • Smoking • NSAID use • Others that may be associated with nonunion	• Psycho-social factors • Back injury-related litigation
Outcome	Nonunion	Patient reported outcomes

Table 2-4   PPO table for a study investigating whether or not procedure type is associated with nonunion in symptomatic patients with lumbar spinal stenosis.

2.4 Summary

- Formulation of a specific, clear, laser-focused, and answer-able study question(s) is a firm prerequisite to planning your study. Someone reading your study question should know precisely what is being evaluated, in whom, and how.

- The framework provided by constructing the PICO table for a treatment or diagnostic study or the PPO table for studies evaluating factors that influence outcomes (eg, risk factors for a poor outcome) helps you conceptualize and specify the primary aspects of your study. Not only does this help you refine your study question and define inclusion/exclusion criteria, it also lays the groundwork for structuring your literature search and focusing on the types of interventions, risk factors, and outcomes that you will need to measure.

- It is worth the time and effort to go through this process as it truly sets the stage for planning and executing the study.

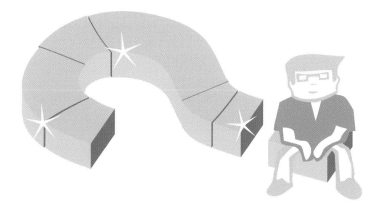

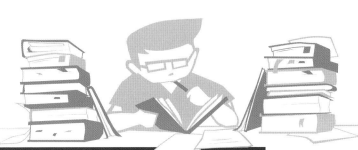

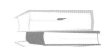

First search, then research.
Getting through the medical literature labyrinth.
Searching PubMed.

3   Constructing a SMART literature search

3.1   Introduction

Now that you have created an answerable, laser-focused question, the next step is to conduct a literature search. The goals of this chapter are to introduce the basic concepts for searching the literature and suggest additional resources. Why is a literature search necessary before planning your study? Here are some of the most important reasons:

- In order to identify any gaps in the evidence that your study will fill (or not), you must know what research has already been published. This may be a requirement for funding and publication of your study.
- Knowing the types of studies that have been published and their findings will help inform your study design. Let us consider three simple scenarios:
  - If your literature search reveals that there have only been many case series on the procedure you want to study, doing another case series may not make a meaningful contribution to the evidence. You should then consider a higher-quality comparative study.
  - If you find ten high-quality randomized controlled trials (RCTs) on the same study question related to efficacy, doing a case series or observational study to answer the same question will likely not enhance the existing evidence. A formal systematic review with or without meta-analysis may be more appropriate.
  - If your search reveals a large number of RCTs that were poorly done and did not report on long-term complications, a well-designed comparative cohort study (or even case-control study) may be the best study design to fill in the gap in the available evidence.

- Information on the outcomes related to your study is necessary in order to determine the sample size (and thus statistical power) needed to effectively answer your question.
- The discussion section of your study will need to include a comparison of the strengths and weaknesses of your own study with previously published works.

3.2   Databases and search engines

Once your study question is formulated and focused, the next step is to identify the best available evidence with which to refine your study question and assist in determining your study design. This begins by identifying the best resources for accessing current information related to your topic.

Electronic databases provide access to the most recent articles with the best evidence to assess therapy, prognosis, and diagnosis. Bibliographic databases contain references to published literature, such as journals and newspaper articles, conference proceedings and papers, reports, government and legal publications, patents, and books. The most common type of literature used for systematic searches is indexed, peer-reviewed literature.

☞ **Peer-reviewed literature is scholarly work that generally represents the original research in a field.**

These articles undergo expert screening before publication to ensure meaningfulness within the context of other research in the discipline and, at least in theory, sound methodology. Another type of literature that may be used, depending on the scope of the topic, is "gray" literature.

☞ **Gray literature refers to material that is not formally published by commercial publishers or peer-reviewed journals, such as reports, fact sheets, white papers, conference proceedings, and other documents from various organizations and government agencies.**

There are many databases available, each with their own focus and limitations. Some of the most common and useful databases and resources are listed in **Table 3-1 and 3-2**.

Database and website	Description	Content
Indexed, peer-reviewed literature		
MEDLINE via PubMed www.ncbi.nlm.nih.gov/pubmed	• National Library of Medicine's (NLM) premier bibliographic database • PubMed is a free search engine maintained by the National Center for Biotechnology Information (NCBI) at the NLM • Contains over 21 million citations • International in scope	• Academic journals covering fields of medicine, nursing, dentistry, veterinary medicine, healthcare system, and preclinical sciences • Much of the literature in biology, biochemistry, and molecular evolution
EMBASE (Excerpta Medica Database) www.embase.com	• Comprehensive biomedical and pharmacological database • Maintained by Elsevier and can be accessed by subscribed users only • Contains over 24 million citations • International in scope	• Active, peer-reviewed journals
Cochrane Reviews www.cochrane.org	• Database comprised of formal, extensive systematic reviews that often contain meta-analysis • Maintained by the Cochrane Collaboration, an international nonprofit organization • Published and hosted by Wiley InterScience • Offers free access to abstracts and some full-length articles, however, most full-text reviews require a subscription or pay-per-view access • Designed to facilitate clinical decision making in healthcare by exploring the evidence for and against the effectiveness and appropriateness of treatments in specific circumstances	• Topics including medications, surgery, technology, and education • Articles are also indexed in PubMed
Cochrane CENTRAL (The Cochrane Central Register of Controlled Trials) www.onlinelibrary.wiley.com	• Collection of databases in medicine and other healthcare specialties • Uses a search interface called OVID	• Focuses on randomized or controlled research studies
AOSpine – EBSS.live www.aospine.org	• Comprehensive database designed to streamline the search process by providing evidence on treatment of spine problems that are organized effectively and graded according to evidence class • Maintained by AOSpine International and requires a paid membership for access	• Summaries of recently published research articles on various topics, including spine therapies, prognoses, and diagnoses

Table 3-1   Common databases and resources providing access to indexed, peer-reviewed literature.

Database and website	Description	Content
Gray literature		
Agency for Healthcare Research and Quality (AHRQ) www.ahrq.gov	• US federal agency responsible for improving the quality, safety, efficiency, and effectiveness of healthcare in the United States • Established evidence-based practice centers (EPC) that develop evidence reports and health technology assessments (HTA) on topics relevant to healthcare organization and delivery issues, specifically those common to and/or significant for the Medicare and Medicaid populations • Provides free online access	• Focuses on synthesizing evidence and facilitating translation of evidence-based research
National Clearinghouse Guidelines (NCG) www.guideline.gov	• Free public resource for evidence-based clinical practice guidelines • Created and maintained by the AHRQ	• Evidence base for guidelines is described • Syntheses of selected guidelines that cover similar topic areas • Expert commentary on issues of interest and importance to the clinical guideline community
International Network of Agencies for Health Technology Assessment (INAHTA) www.inahta.net Center for Reviews and Dissemination (CRD) database www.crd.york.ac.uk	• Database containing information on HTAs, systematic reviews, and economic evaluations from various countries • Managed by the INAHTA Secretariat in collaboration with their UK member Centre for Reviews and Dissemination (CRD) • Free access	• Research including systematic reviews, ongoing and completed trials, questionnaires, and economic evaluations

Table 3-2   Common databases and resources providing access to gray literature.

3.3 A quick search

One of the more user-friendly ways to gain an initial impression of the existing literature on your topic is to start with a search on PubMed, a free bibliographic database search engine that is accessible worldwide. Indexed, peer-reviewed articles will usually give us the best available and most current data. MEDLINE is the primary source of literature for PubMed, which features millions of citations for biomedical articles. PubMed offers various ways to refine and limit your search in order to find exactly what you need from the available literature. Some basics for literature searching will be described in this chapter. However, you may find it helpful to explore the PubMed online training, which contains short tutorials on the essentials of searching, saving, and retrieving articles. The examples and discussion here are intended to give you a basic idea of how to conduct the literature search and get you started. It is beyond the scope of this chapter to describe detailed aspects of the literature search.

A quick way to get an initial idea of the breadth of literature on your topic is to use the Clinical Queries section under PubMed Tools or even a simple basic search on key concepts related to your intended study. Your Patients, Intervention, Comparison, and Outcomes (PICO) or Patients, Prognostic factors, and Outcomes (PPO) table contains key concepts that you can use to perform an initial search. For example, when the concept "lumbar spinal stenosis with interlaminar lumbar instrumented fusion" is typed into the search box in PubMed's Clinical Queries, using the therapy category and specification for a broad search, only one study citation is found and no systematic review citations are found. This may be because we are not searching with the correct concept or there really is nothing published yet on this topic. In contrast, searching for "adjacent segment disease with arthroplasty" results in 44 study citations and nine systematic reviews, indicating perhaps that there is more literature related to this concept.

While the above may be helpful for a quick impression of the existing literature, a more comprehensive and systematic search using more advanced features of PubMed is generally needed. If you have determined that the best study design for your topic may be a systematic review, you will definitely need a more comprehensive and structured search strategy.

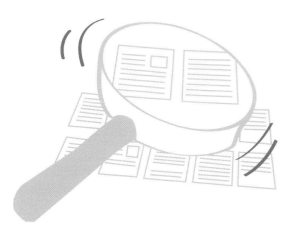

3.4   Structuring a formal search—the basics

Three key elements to formulating a structured search strategy in PubMed are:

- Learning about the controlled vocabulary that is distinctive to MEDLINE, and how to judiciously use key words with it
- Knowing how to combine search terms
- Learning how to narrow or limit the number of citations to those that are potentially most useful

Each of the databases listed in the **Tables 3-1** and **3-2** and other search engines (eg, OVID) have their own structure and methods for searching. Given that PubMed is free, widely available, and user friendly, it is used here to introduce you to these basic concepts. Most of the general concepts described can be applied to other databases and search engines. Consulting their individual guidelines for searching will be important.

3.5   The language of searches in PubMed

Key word searches tell the database to look for a specific word or phrase that appears anywhere in the article title or abstract. Key words are broad and will return articles where the search term is not the main purpose or subject of the article. Key words are useful when you need to make a search more sensitive. A major disadvantage of a key word search is that it does not take into account the meaning of the words used as search terms. If a term has more than one meaning (such as "fixation", which could refer to use of devices to stabilize bone fractures, serologic tests used in immunology, or fixation of nitrogen), irrelevant search results may be generated, depending on how the words are used in the search strategy.

Subject headings are used by databases to index articles into categories as subjects. An article may be given more than one subject heading, but will only be given subject headings that relate to the main purpose or subject of the article. The subject heading may not appear as a word or phrase in the article. Subject headings are useful when you need to make a search more specific. Using subject headings ensures that all items about the same topic have consistent subject headings and can be accessed with one search term. If you're looking for information about the "death penalty" you do not have to search for every word that might be used to describe the death penalty (execution, electrocution, capital punishment, death row, etc). Instead, you can check a list of subject headings in an index or a thesaurus and retrieve all items on the topic with just one search. The most common example of subject heading use is the Medical Subject Headings (MeSH) database and terms. MEDLINE uses this controlled vocabulary to index journal articles and uses automatic term mapping to find MeSH terms when you search. MeSH terms are organized in a hierarchy called a tree, with more specific (narrower) terms arranged beneath broader terms. By default, PubMed includes all narrower terms in the search, which is called "exploding" the MeSH term. Inclusion of MeSH terms enhances and optimizes the search strategy. For example, if you look up the term "Spine" in the MeSH database, it would be positioned in a hierarchy as shown in **Fig 3-1**.

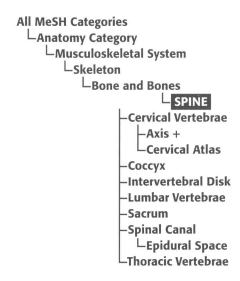

All MeSH Categories
└**Anatomy Category**
　└**Musculoskeletal System**
　　└**Skeleton**
　　　└**Bone and Bones**
　　　　└**SPINE**
　　　　　├**Cervical Vertebrae**
　　　　　│├**Axis +**
　　　　　│└**Cervical Atlas**
　　　　　├**Coccyx**
　　　　　├**Intervertebral Disk**
　　　　　├**Lumbar Vertebrae**
　　　　　├**Sacrum**
　　　　　├**Spinal Canal**
　　　　　│└**Epidural Space**
　　　　　└**Thoracic Vertebrae**

Fig 3-1 MeSH term hierarchy tree.

Therefore, PubMed retrieves every article containing any of the terms located under Spine in the hierarchy. If you want articles on the cervical spine, you may want to drill down and use the term "cervical vertebrae" instead of the broader "spine" term [1].

MeSH, the National Library of Medicine's controlled vocabulary thesaurus, contains over 25,000 descriptors and is updated weekly and reviewed annually. The MeSH thesaurus is used for indexing articles from over 5,000 of the world's leading biomedical journals for the MEDLINE/PubMed database. You can generally only search citations that have been indexed for MEDLINE (92% of the PubMed database) using MeSH terms. Similarly, search queries use MeSH vocabulary to find items on a desired topic. Using MeSH has a number of benefits:

- Allows you to identify and select appropriate MeSH terms for a search and see their definitions
- Facilitates building a PubMed search strategy
- Displays MeSH terms in a hierarchy (MeSH tree) allowing you to broaden or narrow a search
- Permits you to limit MeSH terms to a major concept or topic heading to focus your search
- Allows you to restrict searches to articles focusing only on the broadest MeSH term by choosing not to "explode" a term
- Attaches subheadings for a search creating complex search strategies
- The list of subheadings includes terms paired at least once with a given heading in MEDLINE
- Focuses searches using other types of MeSH terms including publication types, substance names, registry numbers, and pharmaceutical actions

The MeSH database homepage includes brief tutorials on how to search with the database, combine MeSH terms, and apply subheadings and other features of the database.

Learning to effectively use MeSH terms enhances your searching power. One caveat is that since approximately 8% of articles have not been indexed for MEDLINE, it is often wise to use a combination of MeSH terms with the judicious choice of key words.

Other databases may use controlled vocabulary similar to MeSH and some may use MeSH indexing. The basic strategies for building a search are similar but you will need to learn each database's structure separately.

3.6   Combining search terms and wild cards

As an example, suppose we want to answer the following study question: Are the rates of adjacent segment disease lower in adult patients receiving cervical disc arthroplasty compared with patients who received fusion for treatment of symptomatic degenerative disc disease?

We have the basic conceptual components of the PICO approach for that study question, even if we do not have all the specifics:

• Patients: adults with symptomatic cervical degenerative disc disease who are candidates for surgery
• Intervention: arthroplasty
• Comparison: fusion
• Outcome: adjacent segment disease

Utilizing the PICO approach, we structure our search and use at least three sets of search terms:

• Disease/condition
• Intervention
• Cervical spine

In order to find the relevant articles we need to effectively combine these sets of terms by utilizing Boolean logic (ie, OR, AND, NOT). These are the building blocks for structuring your search, and note that they must be capitalized.

How to use OR

OR will combine search terms by finding articles that mention any of the search terms used. For example, **Fig 3-2** illustrates a search for the terms "cat OR dog".

All articles that mention cat and all articles that mention dog will be returned, even if the articles only include one of the search terms specified. OR is most useful when you are combining related or alternative terms as part of a sensitive search strategy.

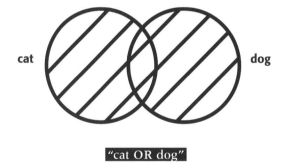

Fig 3-2   Combined search using OR.

How to use AND

AND combines your search terms by only finding articles that mention all of your search terms. For example, **Fig 3-3** shows a search for "cat AND dog" that will only find articles that mention both cat and dog. It will not find articles that mention only cat but not dog or only dog but not cat. Both terms have to be mentioned in the article for it to be included in the results. AND is most useful when you are combining different terms in a search.

How to use NOT

NOT is not available in all search engines, but it is useful to know about it anyway. NOT will eliminate terms from your search. For example, you might want to find an article about cats but not dogs. You could search for "cat NOT dog" as illustrated in **Fig 3-4**. This will find all articles that mention only cat and not those that also mention dog.

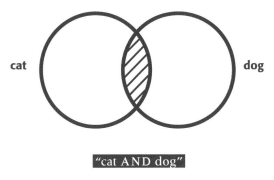

"cat AND dog"

Fig 3-3   Combined search using AND.

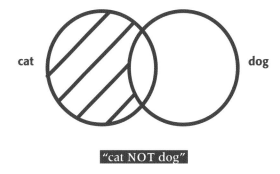

"cat NOT dog"

Fig 3-4   Combined search using NOT.

Taking this one step further, you can combine Boolean operators to further narrow your search. For instance, you could enter "(cat AND dog) NOT bird" as illustrated in **Fig 3-5.**

This will find all articles that mention both cats and dogs, but not those that also mention birds. NOT is useful for focusing the results of your search. You would use NOT to eliminate terms you do not want to include in your results, making your search much more specific.

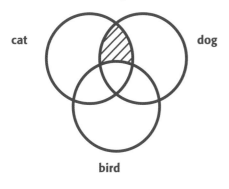

"(cat AND dog) NOT bird"

Fig 3-5   Combined search using both AND and NOT.

3.7   Filters (Limits)

A useful way to limit your results to those that are most relevant is to specify that a term be contained in only the title or abstract. For example, adding [TI] next to a term tells PubMed only to return articles where the term appears in the title. Similarly adding [TIAB] tells it to return only articles in which the term appears in either the title or the abstract.

The "filters" function in PubMed allows you to set commonly used parameters for your query, which may result in more relevant retrieval and help you to refine your search strategy. Depending on which filters you choose to apply, you can restrict your search results to a particular type of study (eg, metaanalysis, clinical trial, comparative study), a particular age group (eg, children 8–12 years old, the elderly), a particular gender, a particular time span, and many other specifications. Your PICO/PPO table again can be a guide.

A word of caution: The indexing in PubMed lags behind the actual appearance of an article in the database. Particularly for newly published articles, this may mean that they may be missed if filters are specified and only MeSH terms are used.

Literature searching is a combination of art and science. It requires practice, intuition, some trial and error, and patience! While there is a basic structure, a set of guidelines, and many tools for assisting one with basic searches, there are also a variety of nuances and advanced techniques that may be required for more specialized searches. For systematic reviews, as an example, extensive searches are required and may take many hours, involving many databases (including those for gray literature), and a combination of advanced search strategies in order to be methodologically sound. Use of personnel with specialized expertise in conducting such searches may provide the best results and be the most resource effective.

3.8 Putting it all together—an example and considerations for study design

The examples in this chapter are intended to illustrate how a search might be structured. They are not intended to provide a comprehensive search on this topic and how various concepts described earlier influence the results of the search.

Table 3-3 lays out the structured literature search for the example study question: Are the rates of adjacent segment pathology (ASP) lower for adult patients receiving cervical disc arthroplasty compared with patients who received fusion for treatment of symptomatic degenerative disc disease?

Search number	Terms	Number of citations returned
#1	adjacent segment disease OR adjacent segment breakdown OR adjacent segment degeneration OR adjacent segment biomechanical consequences OR adjacent segment biomechanics OR adjacent segment motion OR adjacent level disease OR adjacent level breakdown OR adjacent level degeneration OR adjacent level biomechanical consequences OR adjacent level biomechanics OR adjacent level motion	7,034
#2	artificial[TI] OR prosthetic*[TI] OR prosthes*[TI] OR replacement[TI] OR arthroplasty[TI]	126,482
#3	"Prosthesis Implantation"[Mesh] OR "Arthroplasty"[Mesh] OR "Arthroplasty, Replacement"[Mesh] OR "Implants, Experimental"[Mesh]	68,446
#4	#2 OR #3	171,376
#5	"Cervical Vertebrae"[Mesh] OR CERVICAL[TI]	80,865
#6	#1 AND #4 AND #5	148
#7	#6 Filters: Abstract available , Humans, English	112
#8	#6 Filters: Abstract available , Humans, Randomized Controlled Trial, English	20

Table 3-3 Example of a structured literature search.

Note that we used key words for the condition of interest to do a broad search for articles pertaining to the concept of adjacent segment disease using OR in order to be all inclusive. We then turned our attention to searches related to arthroplasty with searches #2 and #3. These provide an example of utilizing the * wild card for truncation, the [TI] specification that articles contain the term in the title, and the use of the MeSH controlled vocabulary. In order to be all inclusive, we used OR to combine these in search #4, noting that we have a lot more citations returned. We then started to focus on the area of the spine that is relevant to our study question. In order to find articles that included concepts related to arthroplasty and adjacent segment disease in the cervical spine, search #6 uses AND to combine the sets of terms to yield 148 articles. For search #7 we added filters, seeking only articles regarding humans which have abstracts and were published in English. Search #8 adds the filter for including only studies indexed as RCTs. You can see that as we added filters, the number of citations decreased, hopefully including the most potentially relevant citations. The purpose and goal of your search influences what filters you use.

The next step is to look at the titles and abstracts to see which citations are relevant and which are not, given your study question and conceptualization outlined in the PICO or PPO table. This gives you a structured, systematic way of assessing what should and should not be included. You can then retrieve the articles for further evaluation.

Using our previous search example, here are some issues to consider when conducting a literature search to inform your study design options and refine your study question:

- With 20 citations related to RCTs, assuming all are relevant, the results may suggest that a systematic review of RCTs may be the best study design to answer the study question.
- On the other hand, after reading the articles and noting their strengths and limitations, you may find that the way that ASP was defined, evaluated, and reported in these studies is not adequate or accurate. A better study comparing the treatments is needed.
- You might also conclude that with the number of comparative studies available, doing a case series with no comparison group would not add to the evidence base.
- You may find that the gaps in the existing literature provide insight into how to better refine your study question to address a more specific aspect of the topic.
- You might find that none of the studies adequately evaluates the risk factors for ASP and that a prognostic study may be warranted.
- You might find that the diagnostic criteria for ASP may have led to erroneous classification of the condition and identified a need for validation or testing of a new method for diagnosing ASP and chose a study design to address this.
- If you are studying the same outcomes reported in the trials, their results can help you determine the sample size needed for your study.

3.9   Summary

- A literature search is necessary to understand the types and quality of evidence that already exist on your topic.

- Using the PICO and PPO approach to specify the major aspects of your study facilitates the literature search.

- A systematic and structured search is suggested for finding the most relevant literature. This allows you to further refine your study question and may provide insight into the best study design that will facilitate a meaningful contribution to the literature.

- The PubMed tutorials are an excellent resource to get you started with a search.

- Use of personnel with specialized expertise in conducting such searches may provide the best results and be the most resource effective if your search is complex and needs to be comprehensive.

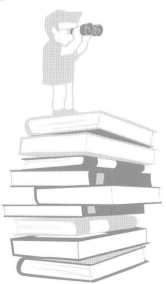

3.10   References

1. **U.S. National Library of Medicine.** National Institutes of Health. PubMed Online Training. [cited November 15, 2011] Available from: http://www.nlm.nih.gov/bsd/disted/pubmed.html.

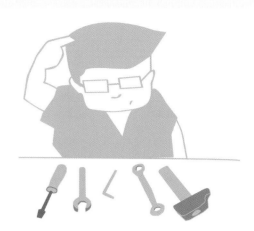

Choosing the right study design is vital. Descriptive versus analytic studies. Overcoming bias is a difficult task.

4   Importance and implications of study design selection

4.1   Introduction

Once you have refined the study question and searched the current body of literature, you must choose a study design that best answers the study question. There are a number of study designs available, but in practice most spine studies fall into a few categories. This chapter provides an overview of those study designs.

Although there are many ways to characterize the various study designs used in spine research, we will do so based on key distinct features [1]. Study designs can be categorized into two major divisions: descriptive and analytic (**Fig 4-1**).

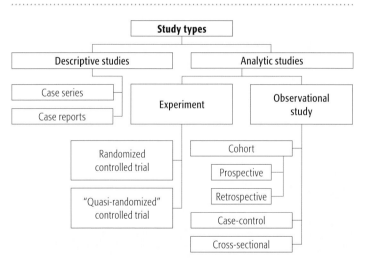

Fig 4-1   Major therapeutic study designs.

Descriptive studies give us a picture of what is happening in a specific patient population. They include case reports and case series, and are carried out generally without stating a specific hypothesis.

Analytic studies are performed in order to answer clinical questions and test hypotheses about how certain interventions affect patient outcome. Analytic studies can further be divided into two main categories: experiments and observational studies.

- Experiments are studies that have some level of random chance used to allocate patients into different treatment groups.
- Observational studies are ones where no formal chance mechanism directs the assignment of patients to a specific treatment group. This can happen when the investigators assign patients to receive different treatments nonrandomly, or when the investigators simply observe the effect of a treatment that was administered without having control over treatment assignment.

4.2   Descriptive studies

Case reports

A case report is a detailed report that describes an unexpected or unusual occurrence. This can include a unique therapeutic or treatment approach, an unexpected association between a disease and symptoms, an unanticipated adverse event, or an unusual combination of signs and symptoms. A case report can help identify new trends, alert others so that they can look for similar occurrences, or provide a basis for a hypothesis that can be tested more formally.

Case series

☞ **A case series is a report of a group or series of patients with a defined disorder treated in a similar manner without a concurrent control group.**

Case series usually contain detailed demographic information on the patients and information on diagnosis, treatment, response to treatment, and follow-up.

Strengths:
- Useful for reporting on relatively rare conditions for which clinical trials may not be feasible (eg, primary spinal tumors)
- As a pilot study to help focus a study question, clarify a hypothesis, determine sample size, or help to determine feasibility
- Useful for introducing new surgical procedures, techniques, or orthopedic devices
- Useful when providing information on safety
- Applicable when the outcome for a new treatment is markedly better than current treatments. This happens when the relative benefit (or risk) for the outcome is very large comparing the new treatment with standard treatments, and the outcomes of standard treatments are well known.

Weaknesses:

- Case series have no concurrent comparison or control group, therefore the effect of a specific treatment cannot be compared to another treatment. In the context of spine surgery, the superiority of a specific surgical procedure cannot be assessed relative to conservative care or to another surgical procedure.
- Case series are often performed retrospectively.

👉 **Retrospective studies are poor at controlling bias because they use existing data that have been recorded for reasons other than research; they are limited to the variables available in the medical records; they are dependent on the accuracy of the prerecorded data; they usually do not provide for blinding of the outcomes assessment; and, in some cases, they rely on a patient's recall for pretreatment clinical status.**

- Case series are often subject to selection bias because the investigator self-selects the cases. For example, consider a case series that included all patients undergoing spinal fusion using a new technique and who had readable follow-up x-rays available. A "good outcome" is one where fusion is demonstrated and the patient has a 30% improvement in pain. In this example, 90 of 130 patients had follow-up x-rays, and thus make up the study population. As illustrated in **Fig 4-2**, 67% of patients had a "good outcome".

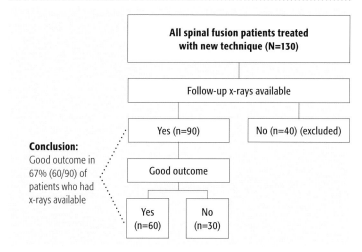

Conclusion: Good outcome in 67% (60/90) of patients who had x-rays available

Fig 4-2   Patients with a "good outcome" among those included in a case series.

4.3   Analytic studies

Now let us suppose that among those patients without x-rays available at follow-up, some did not return because they had problems and decided to see another surgeon, a few moved away from the area, and a few had unreadable x-rays. These patients tended to have worse outcomes (**Fig 4-3**).

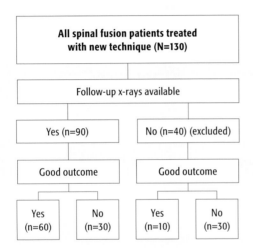

Fig 4-3   Patients with a "good outcome" among those excluded in a case series.

This is an example where selection bias caused an overestimation of the true proportion of those with a "good outcome" which was 54% (70/130), not 67%. As a result of these weaknesses, case series provide a low level of evidence for establishing treatment effectiveness or identifying prognostic factors for good or bad outcomes.

The purpose of conducting an analytic study is to test a hypothesis of whether an "exposure" causes a certain outcome. Exposure is a general term that can refer to an intervention (treatment) or to a risk factor (a characteristic). Interventions are usually modifiable by the investigator, risk factors generally are not. For interventions, all analytic studies described below are available for use. For risk factors, all observational study designs are available, but the randomized controlled trial (RCT) generally is not suitable.

Experiments

Randomized controlled trials

A randomized controlled trial is an experiment in which a formal chance mechanism is used to assign patients to receive an intervention or to serve as a control [1, 2]. Randomized controlled trials generally provide information on how treatments perform under ideal circumstances and evaluate the efficacy of a treatment. Schematically the study design looks like Fig 4-4.

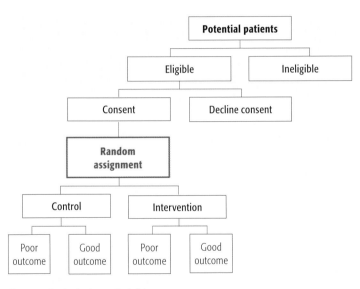

Fig 4-4   Randomized controlled trials.

In this study design, potential patients are screened against a priori inclusion and exclusion criteria. Consenting patients then undergo a formal random allocation process. The random allocation process is made up of two steps:

- Generating an unpredictable random sequence
- Implementing the sequence in a way that conceals the treatments until patients have been formally assigned to their groups

Generating an unpredictable random sequence can be done using a simple random allocation approach. In simple random allocation, treatment assignment is made by chance without regard to prior allocation (ie, it has no memory of the past and it is not discoverable ahead of time). Good methods of generating a random allocation sequence include using a random numbers table or a computer program that generates the random sequence. There are manual methods of achieving random allocation, such as tossing a coin, drawing lots, or throwing dice. However, these manual methods in practice often become nonrandom, are difficult to implement, and do not leave an audit trail [3]. Additionally, concealment may be an issue as there is a possibility that the investigator may alter assignments. Therefore, in general they are not recommended. Procedures to avoid completely include using hospital chart numbers, alternating patients sequentially, assigning by date of birth, and similar schemes.

Concealment is the technique of ensuring that implementation of the random allocation sequence occurs without foreknowledge of treatment assignment. This is distinct from sequence generation. Concealment shields those who enroll patients into a study from knowing the upcoming assignments. In other words, the decision to include or exclude a patient into a trial should be made in ignorance of the upcoming assignment because knowledge of the next assignment could influence whether a patient is included or excluded based on perceived prognosis.

The following are considered adequate approaches to concealed allocation:

- The central randomization technique requires the individual recruiting the patient to contact a methods center by telephone or secure computer after the patient is enrolled.
- Using sequentially numbered, opaque, and sealed envelopes is generally acceptable, but may be susceptible to manipulation [4]. If investigators use envelopes, some suggest that the envelopes receive numbers in advance, are opened sequentially, and only after the participant's names are written on the appropriate envelope. In addition, pressure-sensitive paper inside the envelope should be used to transfer information to the assigned allocation. This can then serve as a valuable audit trail [3].

Strengths:
- Generally considered the strongest design for establishing causation
- Offers protection against confounding, both known and unknown
- Allows direct estimation of incidence (of successful or unsuccessful outcomes)
- Can measure several outcomes in the same study

Weaknesses:
- Often has limited external validity due to strict study inclusion and exclusion criteria (ie, the extent to which the results of the trial are applicable to other populations varies)
- Not suitable for rare outcomes
- Treatment concepts or preferences may change over time
- Can be expensive
- May take several years
- Difficult to study outcomes in the distant future

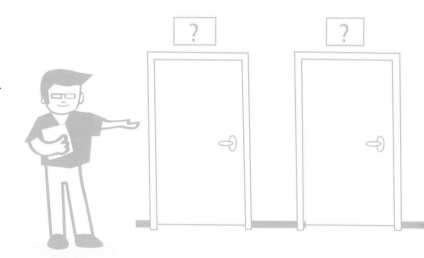

"Quasi-randomized" controlled trial

For a "quasi-randomized" controlled trial, the assignment of the study participants is systematic but not truly random [5]. Schematically this study design is similar to **Fig 4-4** except the assignment is not random. Some believe the term "quasi-random" is unacceptable for describing these trials as they generally yield biased results in part from an inability to conceal allocation [6]. Examples of such designs include assignment by:

- Alternation (or rotation if there are more than two treatment groups)
- Date or year of birth
- Hospital or case record
- Date of presentation or hospital admission

These systematic but not completely random methods suffer from an inability to conceal the treatment assignment and generally allow for biased allocations.

Observational studies
Cohort studies

A cohort study compares outcomes over time between groups with different exposures. In therapeutic studies, these exposures are different treatments. Schematically the study design looks like those of an RCT except that allocation to treatment is not random. They provide information on the effectiveness of a treatment in a more real world setting.

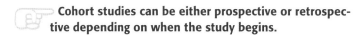 **Cohort studies can be either prospective or retrospective depending on when the study begins.**

Studies that are initiated prior to the occurrence of outcomes are prospective, while those starting after the outcomes have been collected are retrospective. This is illustrated in **Fig 4-5**.

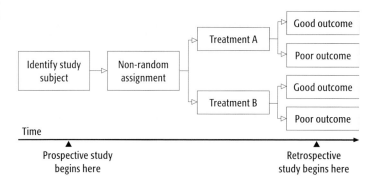

Fig 4-5   Prospective and retrospective cohort studies.

Given that reasons other than chance establish the treatment groups in cohort studies, it is important to consider why participants end up in a particular treatment group. For example, the reason that one patient receives anterior cervical fusion with instrumentation and another receives anterior cervical fusion without instrumentation may be due to a number of factors, such as surgeon training or preference, patient preference, disease severity, intrinsic patient factors (comorbidity, bone health, age, etc), geographic location of the patient, and referral pattern of the primary care practitioner.

Strengths:
- Provides a direct estimation of incidence (successful or unsuccessful outcomes)
- Can measure several outcomes in the same study
- Offers improved external validity compared with randomized trials (ie, the results are likely to apply to a wider range of patients that are treated in real life)

Weaknesses:
- Difficult to control for selection bias and confounding factors
- Not suitable for rare outcomes
- Difficult to study outcomes in the distant future
- Can be expensive and time consuming, particularly prospective cohort studies

While retrospective cohort studies can reduce the cost and shorten the time compared with a prospective cohort study, retrospective studies are limited to the available data. Data collected before conception of a study are often lacking, thus preventing one from studying an important outcome or identifying important demographic information.

Case-control studies

A case-control study is often misunderstood and confused with a retrospective cohort study. A retrospective cohort study identifies groups based on their treatment and then determines their outcome over time. A case-control study identifies groups based on their outcome and then determines which exposure (eg, treatment) they received. **Fig 4-6** illustrates this study design.

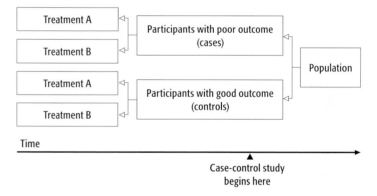

Fig 4-6   Case-control studies.

Case-control studies are used infrequently in surgical disciplines. However, in certain instances, they should be considered.

Strengths:
- Suitable for rare outcomes (since groups are formed on outcomes, the investigator can gather cases from a broad source, such as a registry)
- Can measure multiple exposures in the same study
- Can be relatively inexpensive and quick to conduct

Weaknesses:
- Can be difficult to select the right controls (controls should represent the population from which the cases come)
- Does not provide a direct estimation of incidence (successful or unsuccessful outcomes), but rather provides a relative comparison (a ratio)

Cross-sectional studies

Randomized controlled trials, cohort studies, and case-control studies describe a relationship where an exposure precedes an outcome in time

Cross-sectional studies measure the exposure and outcome at the same time (Fig 4-7). Since exposure and outcome are measured at the same time, it is often unclear which came first.

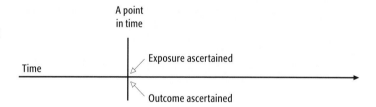

Fig 4-7   Cross-sectional study.

For example, in a cross-sectional study Vogt et al [7] assessed the association between smoking status and low back pain severity among 25,455 patients with information contained in a National Spine Network database. At the initial evaluation the patients' smoking status and symptom severity were gathered. This study found that smokers were more likely to report severe low back pain symptoms than nonsmokers (37% versus 50%). However, the study was not designed to determine which came first: smoking that results in more severe symptoms, or more severe symptoms that lead some to smoke. Data from cross-sectional studies are often obtained by surveys.

Strengths:
- Relatively quick and easy to conduct (no long periods of follow-up)
- Data are collected once
- Multiple outcomes and exposures can be studied
- Good for providing initial information about the associations between exposures and outcomes or for generating hypotheses

Weaknesses:
- May be difficult to determine whether the outcome followed or preceded the exposure in time (ie, cannot determine cause and effect)
- Measures prevalence and not incidence (prevalence refers to the proportion of individuals with a condition at a certain point in time)
- Associations identified may be difficult to interpret
- Often susceptible to bias due to low response
- Misclassification may result if data collected rely on patient recall which may be biased

Alternate study designs

Individuals participating in clinical trials typically have preferences for the treatments under evaluation and may decline to consent to randomization. When treatments cannot be blinded, which is often the case with surgery, patients randomly allocated to their nonpreferred intervention may experience "resentful demoralization", which is a term coined by Cook and Campbell [8]. This describes the resentment and demoralization of people allocated to less than desirable control conditions where they feel deprived of their preferred treatment. This may lead to worse outcomes, either directly (through poor adherence to treatment) or indirectly (through a negative placebo-like effect) [9]. Thus, preferences may introduce bias (ie, reduced internal validity). Other trial designs have been developed to address such problems including the comprehensive cohort design (also known as the Brewin-Bradley design), the 2-stage randomized designs (Wennberg and Rücker designs), and the fully randomized preference trial [10–13].

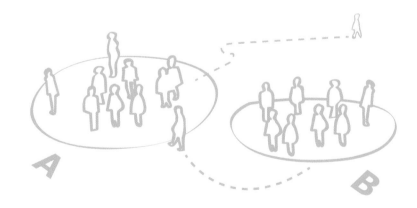

Comprehensive cohort design

In a comprehensive cohort design, patients with strong preferences are offered their treatment of choice, while those without strong preferences are randomized in the conventional fashion. All patients (whether randomized or not) are followed up in the same way as is illustrated in **Fig 4-8**.

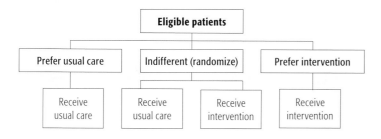

Fig 4-8   Comprehensive cohort design.

Strengths:
• Helps to remove the preference effects from the trial results
• Nonrandomized groups are also followed up to see what happens to people who receive the intervention they desire

Weaknesses:
• Participants with preferences are not randomized exposing parts of the trial to selection bias and making comparisons of these parts of the trial risky
• A high proportion of participants with preferences endangers recruitment to the randomized group
• Since it is not known for sure that preferences will affect outcomes, using this design might result in losing participants from randomization

Comparing the two groups in the randomization cohort allows an estimate of the relative value of the two treatments, but with the added advantage that the groups would not differ in their motivation to follow the specific rehabilitation for the treatment that had been allocated. The influence of motivational factors on outcome of treatment can be studied by comparing usual care with usual care and intervention with intervention between the preferred and randomized groups. If outcomes in preferred groups are significantly better than outcomes in the randomized groups, the motivational factors will be seen as important. If not deemed important, the preferred and randomized usual care and intervention groups can be combined for subsequent analyses.

2-stage randomized design

In the 2-stage randomized design, participants are initially randomized into two groups. In the first group they are offered a choice of treatment and in the second group they are randomly assigned to a treatment. The Rücker design is similar; however, participants randomized to a preference in the first randomization, who do not have a strong preference for a treatment, are randomized a second time to a treatment (**Fig 4-9**).

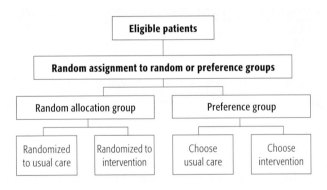

Fig 4-9   2-stage randomized design.

Strengths:

- Helps to remove some of the preference effects from the trial results
- Nonrandomized groups are also followed up to see what happens to people who receive the intervention they desire

Weaknesses:

- The 2-stage randomized design still does not deal with the effects of preference completely. In the randomized group participants still have their preferences, which can affect the outcome of comparison between those two groups.

Fully randomized preference trial

In a fully randomized preference trial, consent and preference are recorded before randomization, and all eligible participants are randomized and treated according to their random assignment (**Fig 4-10**).

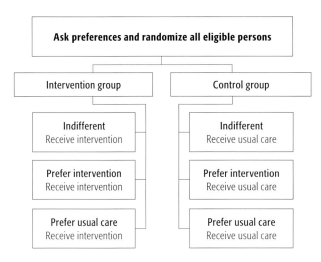

Fig 4-10   Fully randomized preference trial.

Strengths:
- An estimate of the effect of the intervention among participants with and without a preference can be calculated

Weaknesses:
- Participants who have a strong preference for a specific treatment may not consent to the trial

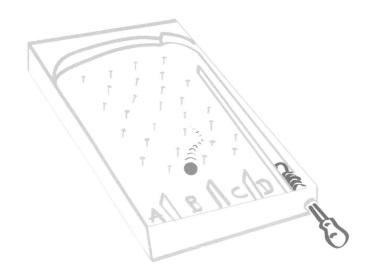

4.4   Summary

- Which study design you choose depends on the study question, and the resources and time available.

- Descriptive studies (case reports or case series) are useful in describing unexpected or unusual occurrences, rare conditions, or new procedures, techniques, or devices. They also are useful in generating or refining a hypothesis.

- Analytic studies are useful in testing hypotheses that compare exposures or treatments.

- Randomized controlled trials are the strongest design for establishing causation and controlling for confounding factors. It helps to limit the bias that comes with the selection of participants for the study. However, other types of bias can enter into any study design, including RCTs.

4.5   References

1. **Koepsell TD, Weiss NS** (2003) *Epidemiologic Methods: Studying the Occurrence of Illness.* New York, NY: Oxford University Press.

2. **Bhandari M, Tornetta P III, Guyatt GH** (2003) Glossary of evidence-based orthopedic terminology. *Clin Orthop Relat Res;* (413):158–163.

3. **Schulz KF, Grimes DA** (2002) Allocation concealment in randomised trials: defending against deciphering. *Lancet;* 359(9306):614–618.

4. **Bhandari M, Guyatt GH, Swiontkowski MF** (2001) User's guide to the orthopedic literature: how to use an article about a surgical therapy. *J Bone Joint Surg Am;* 83–A(6):916–926.

5. **Higgins JPT, Altman DG** (2008) Assessing risk of bias in included studies. *Higgins JPT, Green S (eds). Cochrane Handbook for Systematic Reviews of Interventions.* Chichester: John Wiley & Sons, 187–242.

6. **Moher D, Hopewell S, Schulz KF, et al** (2010) CONSORT 2010 Explanation and Elaboration: updated guidelines for reporting parallel group randomised trials. *J Clin Epidemiol;* 63(8): 1–37.

7. **Vogt MT, Hanscom B, Lauerman WC, et al** (2002) Influence of smoking on the health status of spinal patients: the National Spine Network database. *Spine;* 27(3):313–319.

8. **Cook TD, Campbell DT** (1979) *Quasi-Experimentation: Design and Analysis Issues for Field Settings.* 1st ed. Boston: Houghton Mifflin.

9. **Janevic MR, Janz NK, Dodge JA, et al** (2003) The role of choice in health education intervention trials: a review and case study. *Soc Sci Med;* 56(7):1581–1594.

10. **Brewin CR, Bradley C** (1989) Patient preferences and randomised clinical trials. *BMJ;* 299(6694):313–315.

11. **Wennberg JE, Barry MJ, Fowler FJ, et al** (1993) Outcomes research, PORTs, and health care reform. *Ann N Y Acad Sci;* 703:52–62.

12. **Rücker G** (1989) A two-stage trial design for testing treatment, self-selection and treatment preference effects. *Stat Med;* 8(4):477–485.

13. **Torgerson DJ, Klaber-Moffett J, Russell IT** (1996) Patient preferences in randomised trials: threat or opportunity? *J Health Serv Res Policy;* 1(4):194–197.

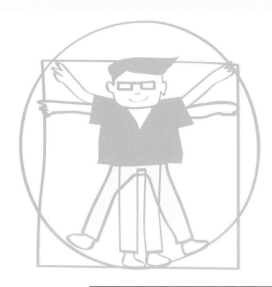

Who, what, when, where, and how to measure.

There's more to measure than outcomes.

Don't collect data that you don't need.

5   Measurements:
the backbone of the study

5.1   Introduction

A study cannot be planned without a well-thought-out, measureable, and clinically meaningful study question or a set of study questions (chapter 2: Constructing a SMART study question). Although study questions should be short and concise, the measurements necessary to address these study questions should be detailed, since they are an integral part of planning a quality research project. It is frustrating to discover in a study report that the stated objectives or study questions were neither answered nor adequately addressed because important measurements were not collected or accounted for at baseline or the outcomes used were not clinically relevant (ie, lacked content validity). Without careful thought and planning, even a study with the best study questions will fail to deliver the results needed to support desired claims, future clinical practice, and ultimately, treatment policy and decision making.

Your choice of measurements is essential to the success of your study. The Patients, Intervention, Comparison, and Outcomes (PICO) or Patients, Prognostic factors, and Outcomes (PPO) table provides you with the general concepts that need to be measured in your study (chapter 2: Constructing a SMART study question). You now need to figure out how to measure or operationalize the data so that they can be collected. In other words, what specifically will you measure using what methods? Studies are primarily about what to measure, when to measure, and how to measure. Methods need to be created for measuring a host of factors, starting with the screening of participants for eligibility and finishing with the most meaningful outcomes of your study. The primary outcomes measurement is the basis for determining sample size and informs the types of statistical analyses that will be necessary. All of these should be carefully thought out a priori and documented in your study protocol. Your study protocol will need to detail specifically what is to be measured, how, when, by whom, and why. It should be clear how the measurements relate to answering your study questions and meeting your objectives.

This chapter reviews the common categories of measurement and provides some of the framework for measurement selection. Later in this chapter you will find a case example on how you might apply the concepts from this chapter to a real-world study scenario.

5.2   Categories of measurement

With regards to measurements, researchers often focus on outcomes. However, measurements from at least four categories are generally needed:

- Baseline factors
- Treatment factors
- Perioperative or immediate posttreatment events
- Outcomes

This chapter briefly covers the first three categories and expands more thoroughly on outcomes measurements. The first three categories may also be considered potential confounding factors when evaluating the association between an exposure and an outcome (chapter 8: Bias reduction). Therefore, a thoughtful selection of potential measurements is paramount to the success of your study.

Baseline factors

All studies require the collection and presentation of baseline patient factors for subjects that meet inclusion and exclusion criteria and are successfully enrolled or included in your study population.

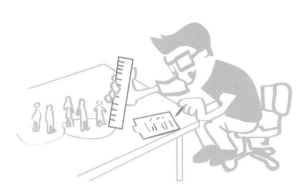

These baseline patient factors help you understand your study population so that you can determine the breadth and scope of your study's generalizability. These factors may simply be descriptive in nature but can also be valuable data points in your analysis. These baseline factors might be considered exposures, risk factors, prognostic factors, predictor variables, potential confounding variables (chapter 8: Bias reduction), explanatory variables, and even effect modifiers. Essentially, they represent the host of factors that each individual patient brings to the study. These factors may influence or be associated with the treatment and outcome. All potential factors should be listed and collected based on a thorough literature review, pilot data (if available), and clinical experience. For prospective studies, these can be built into the data collection forms. For retrospective studies, only variables available in the source data (eg, medical records, registry, administrative database) can be collected. Therefore, those that are not available, yet deemed important, should be listed in the limitations section of the final manuscript. The following list may serve as a general guide for the type of baseline factors to measure:

- Age, gender, education level, hospital, and geographic area
- Disease or diagnosis-specific factors (eg, previous surgery, degenerative disc disease)
- Comorbidities (eg, obesity, diabetes, heart disease)
- Concomitant medications
- General health behavior (eg, smoking, alcohol consumption)
- Socioeconomic or psychosocial variables (eg, litigation, worker's compensation, depression)
- Physical status measurements (these are often outcomes as well but should be measured at baseline to assess change, eg, Visual Analogue Scale (VAS) for pain, Oswestry Disability Index (ODI), Roland-Morris Disability Questionnaire)

- Relevant classification or specific disease severity measures (eg, Kellgren and Lawrence osteoarthritis severity grade, Modic changes, Carragee lumbar disc herniation classification) [1]
- Relevant disease specific measurements (eg, Harris basion axial interval, Power's ratio, Lee x-line method) [2]

Treatment factors

Treatment factors include the primary surgical procedures, additional procedures (eg, bone graft), devices used, and postoperative management strategies, such as nursing procedures (eg, compression stockings), medications, and rehabilitation procedures, depending on the study focus and other outcomes. Most of these items are available in the patient medical records and easy to access. However, they need to be identified before starting the study so that standardized abstraction forms can be created and followed. Postoperative management strategies may be standard operating procedures. However, it is important that these be controlled if necessary (for prospective studies), and detailed in the methods section of your study protocol and the final manuscript in order to ensure that cointerventions are applied equally. Otherwise, bias is possible in a comparison study where treatment groups may not receive the same postoperative management.

☞ **A common problem in many clinical study reports is that too much attention is paid to describing the technique instead of reporting other factors associated with the treatment that may influence the outcome.**

Perioperative or immediate posttreatment events

Perioperative or immediate posttreatment events may influence the outcomes, such as procedure time, blood loss, perioperative or immediate postoperative medications, and immediate postoperative complications. Other events could include the time spent in the hospital and intensive care unit. Most of these items are available in patient records and easy to access. Important factors should be identified before starting the study, since these events may serve as outcomes or as variables that need to be controlled in the final analysis.

Outcomes

Selecting your outcomes measurements is a critical step in research planning. Since study results may lead to recommending a course of treatment for spine care, it is important that they be chosen judiciously. This, however, can be a challenging task. One treatment protocol or intervention may be deemed better than another based on a specific outcome measurement (eg, pain), but not as good based on another measurement (eg, quality of life). A well-designed study that clearly delineates superiority of one treatment over another may provide insufficient evidence or even be harmful if it fails to measure a clinically important outcome. A number of factors need to be considered including:

- Are measurements of the outcome valid and reproducible in the population being studied?
- Are they meaningful to patients?
- Do they provide a meaningful estimate of improvement?
- Do they represent a direct outcome or are they a surrogate for such an outcome?

☞ **Identifying and measuring clinically important outcomes is critical to effective measurement and evaluation of treatment effectiveness. Selecting clinically important outcomes is a challenging task and careful thought is required. The choice of outcomes should tie directly to the study objectives.**

The health status of a population has traditionally been measured in terms of mortality and morbidity rates. Yet, with the epidemiological transition from infectious diseases to chronic diseases (which includes many spine conditions), quantifying health in terms of death and disease rates is seen to be increasingly inadequate [3]. In spine care there are a myriad of potential physiological (eg, bony union) and clinician-based outcomes (eg, range of motion, walking tests) available for use in clinical studies [2]. Depending on the study objective, such measurements may be important but also time consuming and may not represent real function or factors that are important to patients. Complications, however, should always be reported as a measurement of safety [4]. Other measurements from the clinician's perspective should be justified. It is not uncommon for there to be a mismatch between the patient's perception and the clinician's assessment [5]. Therefore, it is increasingly recognized that traditional clinician-based outcome measurements need to be complemented by measurements that focus on the patient's concerns in order to evaluate interventions and identify whether one treatment is better than another [6].

Patient-reported outcomes

The increasing complexity of treatment allocation, acceptability, and utility makes the views of patients more critical in intervention development, evaluation, and health services planning. Emerging patient-reported outcomes (PRO) measurements are doing a better job of measuring aspects of patients' lives that patients themselves consider important. Furthermore, PRO measurements are generally being more carefully developed and tested.

Patient-reported outcomes are questionnaires or instruments that patients complete by themselves or, when necessary, by others on the patient's behalf in order to obtain information in relation to functional ability, symptoms, health status, health-related quality of life (HRQoL), and results of specific treatment strategies.

Interest in PROs has been fueled by an increased recognition of the importance of chronic conditions, where the objectives of treatment are to restore or improve function while preventing future functional decline [7]. Patient-reported outcomes extend beyond traditional clinical efficacy and adverse effects. They represent the patient's perspective on the impact of disease and its treatment on daily functioning and well-being. The Food and Drug Administration (FDA) in the United States has released draft guidance encouraging the use of PROs in clinical trials for new medical products due to the following reasons:

- Some treatment effects are known only to the patient.
- There is a desire to know the patient perspective about the effectiveness of a treatment.
- Systematic assessment of the patient's perspective may provide valuable information that can be lost when that perspective is filtered through a clinician's evaluation of the patient's response to clinical interview questions.

Similar recommendations are being made for health policy decisions. Some have argued that effective policy and planning of healthcare services is dependent on their impact on the individual and their families, underscoring the importance of assessing PROs [8].

Patient-reported outcomes are classified as either general (generic), condition-specific, or patient-preference measurements of HRQoL. General measurements are designed to be used across different diseases and across different demographic and cultural subgroups [9]. They are usually multidimensional and are designed to give a comprehensive and general overview of HRQoL. Spine-specific measurements of HRQoL, on the other hand, focus on aspects of health that are specific to an injury (eg, fractures), disease (eg, spinal stenosis), anatomical region (eg, cervical spine), or population of interest (eg, the elderly). In a recent systematic review by Devine et al [10] (which evaluated the change in condition-specific pain, function, and general quality of life after spine surgery), several validated outcomes instruments that measure a variety of constructs and domains were available to assess the success of treatment for chronic low back pain. Devine et al concluded there is little correlation between the change in pain outcomes and the change in HRQoL outcomes after spine surgery for low back pain, indicating they are measuring different constructs. Pain and functional outcomes instruments were the most responsive to surgery for low back pain and the only outcomes instruments that demonstrated a large effect size. None of the HRQoL tools, including the short form-36 (SF-36), were as sensitive to the treatment. The authors recommended administering VAS for pain and a physical measurement, such as ODI, before and after surgical intervention since these outcomes are the most treatment specific and responsive to change. They recommended against routinely administering an HRQoL measurement or selecting a shorter version (eg, SF-12) in the clinical and research setting to maximize clinical utility, since the measurements are the least responsive to spine surgery. A recent important application of PROs is the use of preference-based outcomes.

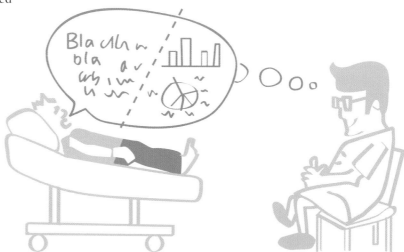

Preference-based outcomes

Due to the increased use and costs for healthcare services, health authorities and policymakers have become interested in the effectiveness and cost-effectiveness of healthcare interventions. Patient-perceived health status is an important healthcare outcome, relevant to patients, surgeons, and policymakers. However, a full discussion of these issues and how they are used in formal economic analyses is beyond the scope of this book. The most common preference-based outcomes measurements are the EuroQol-5D (EQ-5D) and the SF-6D. Both outcome measurements have yet to be tested for validity, reliability, or responsiveness in spine populations. However, the SF-6D was found to be sensitive to changes in the health status of patients with rheumatoid arthritis treated with infliximab [11]. The SF-6D was derived by Brazier et al [12] as a preference-based single index from the SF-36 [13]. The main approach in health economics has been to value health status in a single unit of measurement known as quality-adjusted life years (QALY) or "well years". The index or utility scale ranges from 0 (death) to 1 (full health), and is integrated with survival, so that it is not merely the number of years of life expectancy but also the quality of those years that is considered. The SF-6D was developed to bridge the gap between the SF-36 and the QALY approach. This has resulted in a 6-dimensional health classification. A health state is composed of statements from each of the six dimensions, starting with physical functioning and ending with vitality. A total of 18,000 possible health states are defined this way.

5.3   Selecting outcomes

When selecting an outcome for a clinical study, consider its validity, reliability, responsiveness, and clinical utility (eg, patient and clinician friendliness).

Validity

☞ **Validity is commonly defined as the extent to which an instrument measures what it is intended to measure.**

Since validity is not a fixed measurement, an instrument should be considered valid for use in relation to a specific purpose or set of purposes and in a specific patient population [14]. For example, a valid measurement of disability for patients with cervical myelopathy following laminoplasty cannot automatically be considered valid for use in patients with cervical odontoid fractures. Furthermore, validity cannot be

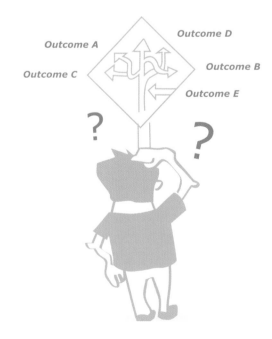

summed up by one concept, but rather can be subdivided into content, criterion, and construct validity. All three are discussed in detail in *Spine Outcomes Measures and Instruments* [15]. The focus of this section is on content validity. If an instrument does not possess the content to support the objectives or claims, its subsequent validity, reliability, and responsiveness are less important. The basis of the content typically starts with an overarching domain. For example, spine outcomes instruments can be divided into the following core domains [16, 17].

- Function
- Pain
- Disability (physical)
- Disability (psychosocial)

Content validity is so important that the International Society for Pharmacoeconomics and Outcomes Research (ISPOR) assigned a task force to report on the importance of content validity, since PROs are used to evaluate the effect of medical products on how patients feel and function [18]. They reported four important threats to content validity:

- Unclear conceptual match between the PRO instrument and intended claim (this can also be applied to a clinical study's objectives)
- Lack of direct patient input into PRO content for the target population in which the claim is desired
- No evidence that the most relevant and important content is contained in the instrument
- Lack of documentation to support modifications to the PRO instrument

When selecting the appropriate PRO for a clinical research study, one must first ask the questions: Does the outcome selected match the intent of the study objectives or study questions? Are the claims I hope to make supported by the outcome selected? If not, a new outcome should be considered. This strikes at the heart of the study's intent. What are you trying to ask, evaluate, or claim? Is it pain relief? Is it function or disability? Is it quality of life? Or is it a combination of these?

Reliability
Reliability is concerned with the consistency of the instrument. In other words, it is the ability to measure something the same way twice. Reliability can be divided into reproducibility and internal consistency.

Reproducibility can be further subdivided into interobserver and test-retest reproducibility, both of which are discussed in more detail in *Spine Outcomes Measures and Instruments* [15]. Internal consistency is a measure of how homogeneous or consistent the questions in the scale are and to what extent they are measuring the same thing. Most instruments use several questions or items to assess a single construct or dimension (eg, pain, disability). This is because several related observations typically produce a more reliable estimate than just one [14]. For this to hold true, the questions all need to be similar, measuring aspects of a single attribute [19]. The end result is that individual questions should correlate highly with each other and with the total score of items in the same scale.

Responsiveness

👉 **Responsiveness, also known as sensitivity to change, is a measure of how well an instrument can detect changes as a result of an intervention [20].**

It is possible for an instrument to be both valid and reliable but not responsive. This is problematic when applying an instrument to evaluate a patient's progress or the effects of a particular treatment. A valid and reliable instrument that does not reflect changes as the patient gets worse or improves is of little clinical or research value.

There is evidence that a statistically significant score change from a validated outcomes instrument does not necessarily mean that the change is clinically important [21–25]. Statistical significance is based on many things, not the least being sample size (chapter 6: Analysis). Therefore, a small change in patients being evaluated may be statistically significant if the sample size in the clinical trial is sufficiently large, yet the change may not represent a large enough clinical benefit to the individual patient. For example, if a study of two antihypertensive drugs finds a statistically significant difference between treatment groups favoring one drug, but the difference in blood pressure is 1 mm Hg, this is not clinically significant. From a clinical perspective, we need to evaluate whether a treatment effect is worthwhile or important when making evidence-based treatment decisions [26]. For research purposes, we need to know the size of the score change that is clinically important in order to estimate necessary sample sizes for future studies.

As a result, there is increasing awareness that responsiveness should include the ability to "measure a meaningful or important change in a clinical state" [27]. The concept of minimal clinically important difference (MCID) has been pioneered in an effort to define the smallest meaningful score change [21, 28–31]. Jaeschke et al [31] defined the MCID as the smallest change that the patient perceives as beneficial. A description of how the MCID is determined and calculated can be found in *Spine Outcomes Measures and Instruments* [15].

Clinical utility

For clinical utility, when considering patient friendliness, the following questions are worth considering [15]:

- Can the instrument be completed in a relatively short time?
- Are the questions clear, concise, and easy to understand?
- Will patients be uncomfortable answering the questions?

With respect to whether an instrument is deemed clinician friendly, the following questions should be considered:

- Is this instrument completed by the staff or self-administered?
- What is the staff effort and cost in administering, recording, and analyzing?
- How much time is required to train the staff in administering the instrument?

5.4 Minimizing bias in outcomes measurements

Minimizing bias in outcomes measurements is best accomplished through the use of valid and reliable outcomes measurements and when the assessor is blinded to the treatment received. It is understandable that in many surgical clinical studies blinding is not possible. In these situations, the assessors of the outcomes should be independent (ie, the evaluator should not otherwise be involved in the design and conduct of the study). Minimizing bias in outcomes measurements is discussed in greater detail in chapter 8: Bias reduction.

5.5 Sample size considerations in outcome selection

Bhandari et al [32] evaluated the impact that outcome selection has on the statistical power in orthopedic trauma trials. This review identified 19,942 patients from 196 randomized controlled trials. Seventy-six of these studies had sample sizes of 50 subjects or less. Among these, 29 studies reported continuous outcomes (eg, SF-36 score) and 47 reported dichotomous outcomes (eg, union or nonunion). Studies that reported continuous outcomes demonstrated significantly greater study power than those that reported dichotomous outcomes. Therefore, when designing small studies ($\leq$ 50 subjects), continuous outcomes will better ensure that adequate study power is achieved compared with dichotomous outcomes. Sample size and power is discussed in more detail in chapter 6: Analysis.

5.6   Why are you collecting the measurements?

Before finalizing your battery of instruments, it is important to put them into a summary table or matrix that lists the measurements and when they will be collected. This broad overview allows you to consider whether you are missing key measurements, measuring them at inappropriate intervals, or more commonly, collecting too many measurements (**Tables 5-1, 5-2**). Whether planning a retrospective medical-record review or a multi-site randomized controlled trial, each of these measurements represents an important piece to the puzzle that needs to be considered in order to ensure that the well-intended and well-conceived study question is answered.

- Does each measurement tie directly or indirectly to the stated objectives or study questions?
- Are there extraneous measurements that do not tie to the objectives?
- Are there unnecessary and redundant measurements that are actually surrogates for what you really want to measure?
- Can we eliminate these?

There is a tendency in measurement selection to behave like a kid in a candy store and collect extraneous data that will never be used.

The "let's collect it now and decide later if we need it" approach has the tendency to backfire and potentially create data that is incomplete or not valid due to the unnecessary burden placed on respondents and researchers.

There are also statistical problems that arise from data mining and multiple testing. Measurements should be conceived a priori, tied directly to study objectives, targeted with a clear purpose for collecting them, and represent a baseline factor, treatment factor, perioperative or immediate posttreatment event, or outcome. Your final choices and the rationale for them should be documented in your study protocol, together with specifics of how and when they will be implemented, before you even begin your study.

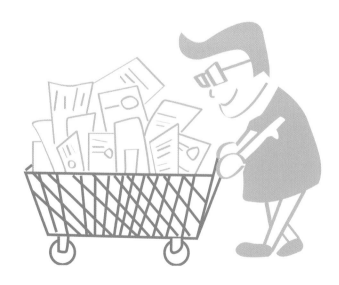

5.7 Case example

....

Comparison of interlaminar lumbar instrumented fusion (ILIF) to posterolateral fusion (PLF): perioperative complications, fusion rates, and clinical outcomes.

Study design: retrospective cohort study

Consider **Tables 5-1** and **5-2** as a checklist for listing all potentially important or clinically relevant measurements by category and then determine if they will be available for your clinical study.

In this example, which is a retrospective cohort study relying on data from medical records, there are several measurements that are not available. This may not invalidate the study design. However, in a cohort study, which does not rely on random assignment (chapter 4: Study design), the inability to account for these factors may bias the results if important unknown factors are unequally distributed between groups. Therefore, the impact should be considered when planning the study. If you choose to pursue it, then this should be acknowledged as a weakness in the discussion of your final manuscript.

Category	Measurement	Availability*
Baseline factors		
Sociodemographic characteristics	Age	X
	Gender	X
	Education level	
	Hospital	X
	Geographic area	X
Disease-specific factors	Duration of symptoms	X
	Previous surgery	X
	Adjacent segment	
	Diagnosis	
Comorbidities	Obesity	X
	Osteoarthritis	X
	Osteoporosis	X
	Diabetes	X
	Heart disease	X
	Other …	
Concomitant medications	Nonsteroidal antiinflammatory drugs	X
	Narcotics	X
	Other …	

Category	Measurement	Availability*
Baseline factors		
General health	Smoking status	X
	Alcohol consumption	
	Other …	
Socioeconomic or psychosocial factors	Pending litigaton	
	Workman's compensation	
	Depression	
	Payor status	
	Other …	
Physical status measurements	VAS pain scale for leg and back	X
	ODI	
	SF-36	
Disease severity measurements	Preoperative sectional area of lumbar canal as seen on MRI	X
	Walking tolerance testing	

Table 5-1   Example checklist matrix of important baseline factor measurements for the ILIF to PLF comparison study.
*An "X" indicates that the measurement is available. If blank, then we consider it important but unavailable.

Category	Measurement	3 months	6 months	12 months
Baseline factors				
Treatment factors	Use of allograft	X		
	Use of autogenous iliac crest bone graft	X		
	Use of instrumentation	X		
	Surgical level	X		
Perioperative factors	Medical complications	X		
	Cardiopulmonary factor	X		
	Gastrointestinal (ileus) factor			
	Surgical complications			
	Neurological change			
	Hardware failure			
	Dural tear			
	Blood loss			
Clinician-based outcomes	X-rays: flexion and extension	X	X	X
	CT scan			
Patient-reported outcomes	VAS pain scale for leg	X	X	X
	VAS pain scale for back	X	X	X
	ODI		X	X
	SF-36		X	X

Table 5-2 Example checklist matrix of measurements (treatment, perioperative, and outcomes), availability, and frequency of data collection for the ILIF to PLF comparison study.

* An "X" indicates that the measurement is generally available. If blank, then we consider it important but unavailable. In any study, particularly a retrospective study, there is always the possibility of missing or unrecorded data. This should be reported in the results section of your study.

5.8   Summary

- A study is not well-planned if it does not include careful consideration and selection of appropriate measurements. Measurements must be directly linked to study objectives and hypotheses, and include baseline factors, treatment factors, perioperative or immediate posttreatment events, and outcomes. Not accounting for these factors may lead to bias in treatment comparisons where an unequal distribution of factors exists. Not selecting appropriate outcomes measurements may lead to results that do not support the intended claims or objectives of the study.

- When selecting outcomes measurements, it is paramount that you consider the appropriate PROs since policymakers, regulatory bodies, and patients' rights groups are requiring inclusion of the patient's perspective.

- When selecting a PRO instrument for a clinical study, consider its validity, reliability, responsiveness, and clinical utility (eg, patient and clinician friendliness). The most important consideration is content validity. Once measurements with appropriate content are selected, then other aspects of validity, reliability, and responsiveness should be considered.

- The MCID concept has been pioneered in an effort to define the smallest meaningful score change. When selecting an outcome, ensure that you measure it at baseline and follow up so that such a change can be calculated. Perform a review of the literature for the MCID with respect to the measurement and population of interest.

- Be careful not to select too many measurements. While you want to make sure that important factors are accounted for, consider also the burden on patients and clinicians. Meeting with your study team to review a full matrix of measurements over time will go a long way in making sure you have collected the most important measurements without overdoing it prior to constructing your case report forms and data collection documents.

- The case example in this chapter provides an example of how to go about selecting appropriate measurements for your clinical study during the planning phase. **Tables 5-1** and **5-2** are examples that should be included in your study protocol.

5.9   References

1. **Chapman JR, Dettori JR, Norvell DC** (eds) (2009) *Spine Classifications and Severity Measures.* Stuttgart New York: Thieme Publishing.

2. **Chapman JR, Dettori JR, Norvell DC** (eds) (2012) *Measurements in Spine Care.* Stuttgart New York: Thieme Publishing.

3. **Goldstein NE, Lynn J** (2006) Trajectory of end-stage heart failure: the influence of technology and implications for policy change. *Perspect Biol Med;* 49(1):10–18.

4. **Andersson GB, Chapman JR, Dekutoski MB, et al** (2010) Do no harm: the balance of "beneficence" and "non-maleficence". *Spine;* 35 Suppl 9:S2–8.

5. **Davidson P, Cockburn J, Daly J, et al** (2004) Patient-centered needs assessment: rationale for a psychometric measure for assessing needs in heart failure. *J Cardiovasc Nurs;* 19(3):164–171.

6. **Koeberle D, Saletti P, Borner M, et al** (2008) Patient-reported outcomes of patients with advanced biliary tract cancers receiving gemcitabine plus capecitabine: a multicenter, phase II trial of the Swiss Group for Clinical Cancer Research. *J Clin Oncol;* 26(22):3702–3708.

7. **Patrick DL** (2003) Patient-Reported Outcomes (PROs): An Organizing Tool for Concepts, Measures, and Applications. *Quality of Life Newsletter;* 31:1–5.

8. **Chang S, Gholizadeh L, Salamonson Y, et al** (2011) Health span or life span: the role of patient-reported outcomes in informing health policy. *Health Policy;* 100(1):96–104.

9. **McSweeny AJ, Creer TL** (1995) Health-related quality-of-life assessment in medical care. *Dis Mon;* 41(1):1–71.

10. **Devine J, Norvell DC, Ecker E, et al** (2011) Evaluating the correlation and responsiveness of patient-reported pain with function and quality-of-life outcomes after spine surgery. *Spine;* 36 Suppl 21:S69–74.

11. **Russell AS, Conner-Spady B, Mintz A, et al** (2003) The responsiveness of generic health status measures as assessed in patients with rheumatoid arthritis receiving infliximab. *J Rheumatol;* 30(5):941–947.

12. **Brazier J, Roberts J, Deverill M** (2002) The estimation of a preference-based measure of health from the SF-36. *J Health Econ;* 21(2):271–292.

13. **Conner-Spady B, Suarez-Almazor ME** (2003) Variation in the estimation of quality-adjusted life-years by different preference-based instruments. *Med Care;* 41(7):791–801.

14. **Fitzpatrick R, Davey C, Buxton MJ, et al** (1998) Evaluating patient-based outcome measures for use in clinical trials. *Health Technol Assess;* 2(14):1–74.

15. **Norvell DV** (2007) Quality outcomes measures. *Chapman JR, Hanson HB, Dettori JR, et al (eds), Spine Outcomes Measures and Instruments.* Stuttgart New York: Thieme publishing, 17–30.

16. **Hansen BP** (2007) Choosing the right outcomes instrument. *Chapman JR, Hanson HB, Dettori JR, et al (eds), Spine Outcomes Measures and Instruments.* Stuttgart New York: Thieme publishing, 9–11.

17. **Chapman JR, Norvell DC, Hermsmeyer JT, et al** (2011) Evaluating common outcomes for measuring treatment success for chronic low back pain. *Spine;* 36 Suppl 21:S54–68.

18. **Rothman M, Burke L, Erickson P, et al** (2009) Use of existing patient-reported outcome (PRO) instruments and their modification: the ISPOR Good Research Practices for Evaluating and Documenting Content Validity for the Use of Existing Instruments and Their Modification PRO Task Force Report. *Value Health;* 12(8):1075–1083.

19. **Streiner DL, Norman GR** (1995) *Health Measurement Scales: A practical guide to their development and use.* 2nd ed. Oxford: Oxford University Press.

20. **Wassertheil-Smoller S** (1995) Mostly about quality of life: A Primer for Health and Biomedical Professionals. *Biostatistics and Epidemiology.* 2nd ed. New York: Springer-Verlag, 147–155.

21. **Beaton DE** (2000) Understanding the relevance of measured change through studies of responsiveness. *Spine;* 25(24):3192–3199.

22. **Bombardier C, Kerr MS, Shannon HS, et al** (1994) A guide to interpreting epidemiologic studies on the etiology of back pain. *Spine;* 19 Suppl 18:2047–2056.

23. **Deyo RA, Diehr P, Patrick DL** (1991) Reproducibility and responsiveness of health status measures. *Statistics and strategies for evaluation. Control Clin Trials;* 12 Suppl 4:142–158.

24. **Deyo RA, Patrick DL** (1995) The significance of treatment effects: the clinical perspective. *Med Care;* 33 Suppl 4:AS286–291.

25. **Epstein RS** (2000) Responsiveness in quality-of-life assessment: nomenclature, determinants, and clinical applications. *Med Care;* 38 Suppl 9:II 91–94.

26. **Hägg O, Fritzell P, Nordwall A, et al** (2003) The clinical importance of changes in outcome scores after treatment for chronic low back pain. *Eur Spine J;* 12(1):12–20.

27. **Liang MH** (2000) Longitudinal construct validity: establishment of clinical meaning in patient evaluative instruments. *Med Care;* 38 Suppl 9:II 84–90.

28. **Hays RD, Woolley JM** (2000) The concept of clinically meaningful difference in health-related quality-of-life research. *How meaningful is it? Pharmacoeconomics;* 18(5):419–423.

29. **Testa MA** (2000) Interpretation of quality-of-life outcomes: issues that affect magnitude and meaning. *Med Care;* 38 Suppl 9:II 166–174.

30. **Wells G, Beaton D, Shea B, et al** (2001) Minimal clinically important differences: review of methods. *J Rheumatol;* 28(2):406–412.

31. **Jaeschke R, Singer J, Guyatt GH** (1989) Measurement of health status. *Ascertaining the minimal clinically important difference. Control Clin Trials;* 10(4):407–415.

32. **Bhandari M, Lochner H, Tornetta P III** (2002) Effect of continuous versus dichotomous outcome variables on study power when sample sizes of orthopedic randomized trials are small. *Arch Orthop Trauma Surg;* 122(2):96–98.

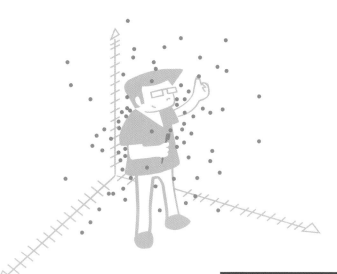

Clean your data set.
Design a SMART analysis plan.
Quality planning ensures proper execution.

6   Analysis: basic statistical methods and principles

6.1   Introduction

A SMART analysis plan should build upon the concepts presented in the previous chapters. The analysis plan is an integral part of the overall study protocol and should be developed at the beginning of the study. Having identified your study questions, study design, and measurements, you should have at least a conceptual idea of how the data are to be analyzed before collecting it. This ensures that your abstraction forms, questionnaires, and study execution plans will gather the appropriate data necessary for the analysis.

Analysis is the consideration of everything from data quality, description, and characterization of the study population to the analytical statistics performed and their correct interpretation. The need for the highest level of data quality is consistent across all study designs. Each study question should have a corresponding analysis plan. A protocol for your study, which includes a statistical analysis plan established a priori, serves as a reference for all those involved in the study and facilitates the writing of the study manuscript. Protocols, grants, and manuscripts that present the analysis plan for each objective are the easiest to understand and execute, and have the greatest credibility. A well-thought-out analysis plan is required for a grant proposal.

The principles set forth in this chapter will assist you in the basics of planning the size of your study, describing your subject populations, and dissecting your study objectives so that you can select the appropriate statistical tests for answering the study questions. This chapter does not go into detail on data collection and monitoring procedures, basic statistical concepts, or definitions, such as median, mean, standard deviation (SD), interquartile range (IQR), or normal and nonnormally distributed data patterns. However, we will apply some of these principles in this chapter. Discussion of sophisticated analysis methods is also beyond the scope of this book.

☞ **This chapter is not going to make you a biostatistician. Its primary purpose is to ensure that you understand the importance of properly designing your analysis plan up front and that it matches each of your study objectives. Its secondary purpose is to expose you to various methods used in data analysis so that you are familiar with the various tools available to you.**

Your SMART analysis plan should include the following components:

- A restatement of your study questions and study design
- A firm understanding of the measurement variables used to answer your study questions
- Power and sample size calculations based on your primary objectives and primary outcomes
- A plan for developing data-collection forms and a database that allows you to execute your analysis plan seamlessly after finishing your data-collection efforts
- An analysis plan for each study question or objective. This begins first with how to handle the descriptive data and then a specific analytical plan for each study question if you are making treatment comparisons or assessing risk factor associations

6.2   Understanding your measurement variables

Measurements are usually labeled as categorical (qualitative) or continuous (quantitative). Categorical data (nominal or ordinal) are counts of the number of participants or observations in each category. These data are often described with percentages or other ratios (eg, rates). Common measurements in spine outcomes research include union and complication rates following surgery. Continuous data are data that, when graphed, form a distribution of values along a continuum. Distributions that form a bell-shaped curve are said to be approximately normally distributed, while all other distributions are non-normally distributed. Approximate normal distributions should be accompanied by a mean and SD, while non-normal distributions are better described by a median and IQR. Mean and median measures indicate where on the continuum the data tend to cluster. The SD or IQR describe the spread or variability of the data over the continuum, respectively. An example of both a categorical and continuous outcome that can be found in one outcomes measurement is the low back pain outcomes score (LBOS) [1]. The LBOS is divided into 13 subscales ranging from current pain to leisure activity. The total score is based on a 75-point scale. Since a person could receive a score between 0 and 75 points, this score can be thought of as a continuous outcome. On the other hand, the authors of the score have also divided it into four potential outcome categories:

- Excellent: ≥ 65
- Good: 50–64
- Fair: 30–49
- Poor: 0–29

These arbitrary divisions create an ordinal categorical variable (ie, there is an order or hierarchy). Furthermore, it is not uncommon for authors to take categorical scores like these and divide them into "Good" and "Poor" outcomes (eg, < 50 = Poor, ≥ 50 = Good). This is still a categorical variable, but is now called a dichotomous (or binary) outcome. Dichotomous outcomes are easier to work with in an analysis, since they allow for the calculation of rates and relative risks, which will be described later. Care must be taken to justify such arbitrary divisions. Ideally, for most outcomes, cut points should be set a priori and not based on a look at the data to determine what may seem most advantageous for the hypothesis to be tested. The type of data influences the types of analyses and statistical tests that are done.

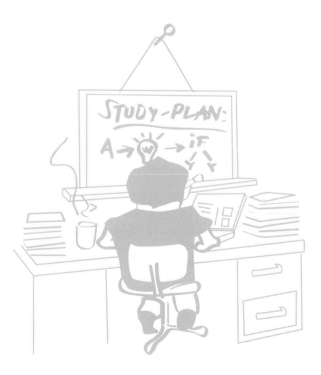

6.3   Power and sample size calculations

For a study to have a reasonable chance of answering its study questions, there must be enough subjects. Before embarking on any data collection, you should first develop a power analysis to best estimate how many subjects you will need in your study to answer the study questions and achieve the study objectives. For a case series (ie, one group) that is evaluating the safety of a treatment, the sample should be large enough to give a reasonably small standard error for the point estimate (eg, complication rate). For a comparison study (ie, randomized controlled trial, cohort study, case-control study), a power calculation determines how many subjects are needed in each group to have enough power (typically 80%) in order to detect a statistically significant difference between two groups. For a prospective study, this will help you determine how long your recruitment period should be based on the number of sites enrolling and what you know about the potential number of patients being treated for the condition of interest. For a retrospective study, this will help you determine how far back you will need to go in extracting data from your source (eg, medical records or registries). When conducting a sample size calculation, you need to answer the following questions:

- What is your study design? Case series? Randomized controlled trial? Cohort or case-control study?
- What are the primary outcomes used to address the objectives?
  - Is it a rate or proportion?
  - Is it the mean of a measurement?
  - Is it a summary score based on a validated instrument?
  - Is it an ordered scale?
  - Is it a survival time?

- What measure of effect is planned based on your primary outcomes? Means? Odd ratios? Relative risks?
- What values are estimated for rates, scores, or times for each treatment group? (Past literature or your own pilot data, if it exists, would help answer this question.)
- How large a difference would be considered clinically meaningful? (This difference may be available in the literature based on the outcome measurement you have selected. It may have to be based on clinical judgment.)
- For the primary outcome measurement, what are the estimated SDs (or other measurement of variability) for each group? (This can be identified in the past literature or your own pilot work. Sometimes this has to be estimated.)

In summary, for performing a sample size calculation you will typically need an estimated rate or mean for the outcome in each treatment group (or estimated clinically meaningful difference) and the corresponding SDs. You will also need to select the significance level (conventionally .05) and the power (typically 80%).

- **Statistical significance relates to how likely the observed effect is due to chance (ie, sampling variation).**
- **Clinical significance relates to the magnitude of the observed effect that is clinically meaningful. A statistically significant result may or may not be clinically meaningful.**
- **Power refers to the ability of a study to statistically detect a true difference between study groups.**

It is possible that one treatment is truly superior to another, yet the study may result in statistically insignificant results. This will occur if the sample size is too small to detect differences in treatment effectiveness. This indicates a problem with the power of the study. This also highlights why it is important

that you describe your sample size calculations to justify your recruitment goals. The sample size needed depends on how frequently the outcome of interest occurs, if you are working with an event or dichotomous outcome. For example, if one is evaluating nonunion for a spinal fusion procedure, and the nonunion rate is 1%, then a study that includes 1,000 patients will yield only 10 patients with nonunion. In this case, 1,000 patients are not enough. On the other hand, if estimated rates are higher, for example 10–20%, then sample size requirements are not so steep.

Keep in mind that the correct interpretation of the results of statistical testing is as important as applying the correct statistical methods. This goes beyond looking at the P value! The P value only assesses the extent to which an observed affect may be due to chance. You may recall the concepts of type I and II errors. In simple terms, a type I error occurs when the results show that a difference exists, but in reality there is no difference. Therefore, lowering the amount of acceptable error would reduce the chances of a type I error (eg, using $P = .01$ instead of $P = .05$). Lowering the amount of acceptable error, however, also increases the chances of a type II error, which refers to the acceptance of the null hypothesis when in fact the alternative is true. Therefore, the greater the chances of a type I error, the less likely a type II error will occur, and vice versa.

Table 6-1 demonstrates that one would need a sample size of 141 patients to show a difference in 10% (eg, 5% versus 15%), comparing treatment groups resulting in a nonunion, assuming 80% power and $P < .05$. Different sample sizes for different scenarios can be estimated from this table. It is a good idea to present your sample size estimates in a table similar to **Table 6-1**.

There are software programs available for download that will calculate sample size requirements (such as the PS: Power and Sample Size Calculation program), as well as web-based programs (such as the program available on the MGH Biostatistics Center website). These programs are user-friendly and allow you to either calculate a sample size estimate from a given level of power, or calculate the level of power for a given sample size. It is generally a good idea to make calculations for a range of estimates in order to protect yourself from relying on a single value as is illustrated in **Table 6-1**.

		Power		
	90%	**80%**	**70%**	**60%**
0.125	106	80	63	50
Difference in proportions **0.100**	188	**141**	111	88
0.075	371	278	219	174
0.050	918	686	540	429

Table 6-1   Hypothetical sample size calculations based on a difference in rates of nonunion between treatment groups.

Once you have figured out your sample size, you need to consider whether a sample of this size is possible. Often we overestimate the number of subjects we can recruit or obtain for a particular study. Careful planning and consideration help you strategize and ultimately decide if your study is feasible and whether you need to consider a different study question, a different measurement, or a longer period of recruitment (for a prospective study) or data extraction (for a retrospective study), or even a different study design.

6.4   Developing your data collection forms and database

If you have clear objectives, measurements that map directly to these objectives, a pre-determined analysis plan, and a clean data set, the analysis should fall right into place. Not only should it be fairly straightforward, but also should be a reward for a job well done.

Although this book focuses primarily on study planning, there is an important overlap in the planning of your data collection and analysis efforts, and how you execute them. Therefore, this chapter briefly discusses data planning and execution. It is critical to develop a complete set of data collection forms that have been vetted by your entire study team. It would be unfortunate to realize part way through your data collection effort (retrospective or prospective) that you have omitted some important data elements. This often requires an institutional review board modification and duplicate efforts to retrieve these data. Do your due diligence up front and come to an agreement with all investigators before starting. When collecting data, you should screen it for accuracy, identifying nonsensical and missing values as soon as possible. Inaccurate or missing data should be queried on a regular basis. Waiting until all data are collected often leads to data issues that are not resolved and possibly the inability to collect or correct necessary data. When performing retrospective studies, similar principles apply. It is important to find the source of the data (eg, electronic medical records, radiology reports) when queries are necessary. There is a tendency to rush into the analysis before the data set is adequately prepared for such purposes. It is critical to generate as clean of a data set as possible with accurate variables and the fewest missing data points before starting the analysis.

Creating a clean data set begins with the planning phase of your study.

> 👉 **Clean data speaks to both data quality and functionality. The three critical aspects to data quality are accuracy of the data, a plan for minimizing and handling missing data, and addressing and correcting nonsensical data.**

The accuracy of the data starts with the source. The source can be anything from medical records, laboratory or radiology reports, or even the patients if the data are obtained through self-report questionnaires. Ensuring accuracy requires that due diligence be done and data collection forms match the source of the data. The full process of data monitoring and auditing is beyond the scope of this book; however, the basic principles are simple to apply. Appropriate checks and balances should be put in place to ensure the data you are entering into your database are accurate. This can be done by periodically doing a full or partial audit of your data collection forms against the source data. This is particularly important for key explanatory or outcomes variables and measurements. For example, if you are interested in the effects of smoking on spine fusion rates, you should make sure that all subjects in your data who are classified as smokers are in fact smokers and all subjects' fusion status is verified from the source documentation.

Once you are confident that the data is accurate, it can be entered into the database. The next step is to investigate whether you have missing or nonsensical values. This can be done by reviewing all the data in a spreadsheet format, which can be challenging when there are many subjects and variables in your data set. The naked eye has a tendency to miss things. Therefore, we recommend transferring the data into a statistical computer program that can inspect each variable for missing values and ranges.

Data functionality has to do with the suitability of the data within your database. In other words, in order to evaluate your data, it has to be in a form that is suitable for statistical analysis. For example, data analysis software operates best when the variable names are short and simple. A data dictionary with the variable name and what it represents is the best way to make sure there is a link between the simple form of the variable and the actual meaning. In addition, the values for each variable for each subject should be a number and not text. The data fields for gender, for example, should not read "male" and "female" but rather as a numerical value, such as "0" and "1" (**Table 6-2**). The data dictionary will break this code (**Table 6-3**). Furthermore, categorical outcomes such as "Poor", "Fair", and "Good" should not be entered as text but rather as numbers such as "0", "1", and "2".

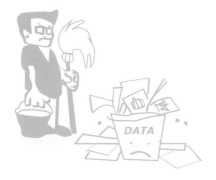

ID	Gender	Fusion	Smoking	LBOScon	LBOScat
1001	Female	Yes	Current	25	Poor
1002	Female	No	Current	57	Good
1003	Male	Yes	Former	70	Excellent
1004	Male	No	Never	33	Fair

Table 6-2   An example of a data format that will not work.

There is never a reason to have text in a data field unless it is an open-ended question. However, text fields are not recommended as you cannot analyze them. Even answers to questions should be given numbers in the database so that frequencies can be generated. The data dictionary will always clarify what the numbers mean.

Data format

ID	Gender	Fusion	Smoking	LBOScon	LBOScat
1001	1	1	2	25	4
1002	1	0	2	57	2
1003	0	1	1	70	1
1004	0	0	0	33	3

Data dictionary notations

Gender	0 = Male	1 = Female		
Fusion (by 6 months)	0 = No	1 = Yes		
Smoking (status at surgery)	0 = Never smoked	1 = Former smoker	2 = Current smoker	
LBOScon (value for continuous form of the LBOS score)	Minimum value = 0	Maximum value = 75		
LBOScat (category of LBOS score based on established cut points)	1 = Excellent (>65)	2 = Good (50–64)	3 = Fair (30–49)	4 = Poor (0–29)

Table 6-3 An example of a data format and data dictionary that will work.

Once you believe your data are accurate, you have recovered all missing data that is possible, the values are within acceptable ranges, and the data are functional, you have a clean data set ready for analysis.

6.5 Analysis plan

Most analyses are divided into descriptive and analytical statistics, which should be clearly described in the methods section of your study. Both types of statistics will likely be used in your clinical study. Descriptive statistics are most frequently used to provide general information about the patients and factors that may be related to outcomes. In one sense, they set the stage for some of the analytical methods (such as control for confounding) that may be needed to ensure the most accurate estimate of a study treatment effect. Analytical statistics allow for evaluation of treatment effects and the associations between factors. Both may involve tests of statistical significance. A helpful table for choosing the appropriate statistical test can be found in **Table 6-5**.

Descriptive statistics

A prospective study allows you to collect all known and suspected potential confounders. For retrospective studies, you are limited to what has already been collected and often do not have access to factors that likely influence outcome (eg, smoking status).

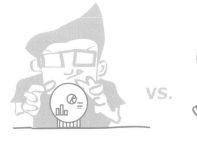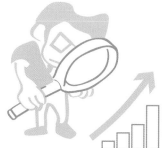

Descriptive statistics are used to simply describe the data you have collected. These data are typically presented in the first table of your manuscript. There should be a clear explanation in the analysis section of your analysis plan as to how you will report these data (eg, categorical and continuous measurements). Descriptive statistics are important for the following reasons:

- They enable you to determine the comparability of study groups at baseline and evaluate the likelihood of any selection bias or confounding (chapter 8: Bias reduction).
- They enable you to present all important factors that may influence outcome. When an analysis cannot include all known or suspected confounders, the estimate of treatment effects may be biased. This is known as an omitted variable or residual confounding bias and is often a problem in retrospective studies. When known potential confounders cannot be included in an analysis, you should acknowledge this as a limitation and describe the anticipated effect.
- The baseline characteristics of the study population can help in determining the generalizability and external validity of the results to other patient populations.
- Baseline scores for pain, function, and quality of life measurements should be presented, especially when used as an outcome or associated with the outcome of interest. The absolute scores at follow-up are often associated with the scores prior to treatment.
- Finally, the descriptive tables presented in a study report typically should describe all enrolled patients. This can allow you to determine the extent of loss to follow-up, when not explicitly stated. (You need to keep track of your loss to follow-up. At the end of the day, the numbers for screened, eligible, enrolled, and lost subjects should add up.)
- Descriptive analyses are best described as univariate analyses (**Table 6-4**).

☞ **As all research is performed on samples of subjects, there is always a possibility, at least in theory, that the results observed are due to chance only and that no true differences exist between the compared treatment groups. Statistical tests help us sort out how likely it is that the observed difference is due to chance only.**

Analytical statistics

The purpose of analytical statistics is to report the effects of treatment and risk factors for specific outcomes. These rely on the testing of statistical hypotheses that are established a priori during the study question phase (chapter 2: Constructing a SMART study question). The testing of a statistical hypothesis (sometimes called testing of statistical significance) is important when using outcomes measurements to declare that a treatment is safe or superior. Statistical tests aim to distinguish true differences and associations from chance.

Commonly, we use an arbitrary test threshold value (eg, alpha = 0.05) to distinguish results that are assumed to be due to chance from the results that are due to other factors. However, we will be wrong one out of 20 times. If the probability that the results are due to chance is less than the threshold value ($P < .05$), we assume the differences are due to these other factors (eg, true differences in treatment effects). Choosing the correct statistical test to compare your outcomes depends on the study design, the types of outcome variables you have collected (**Table 6-4**), and for continuous variables, their distribution (normally or non-normally distributed).

Bivariate analysis

In order to better understand the initial associations between factors in the data, one should consider a bivariate analysis. This is a helpful analysis to conduct prior to more sophisticated methods like regression. Such an analysis allows you to assess the distribution of individual variables and their impact on outcomes, which will lead to a more relevant and strategic development of a statistical model. If explanatory measurements are not equally distributed between study groups and are associated with the outcome of interest, they must be controlled for (chapter 8: Bias reduction). Bivariate analysis allows you to inspect these possibilities in preparation for more sophisticated regression analyses (**Table 6-4**).

Univariate analysis	Bivariate analysis
• Involves a single variable	• Involves two variables
• Does not deal with causes or associations	• May deal with causes or associations
• The purpose is to describe variables	• The purpose is to explain the relationship between variables
• Central tendency—mean and median • Dispersion—range, variance, maximum, minimum, quartiles, SD • Frequency distributions • Bar graphs, histograms, pie charts, line graphs, box-and-whisker plots	• Analysis of two variables simultaneously • Correlations • Associations, causes, explanations • Cross tabulations evaluating the association between two variables • Examining the association between independent and dependent variables (not controlling for other variables)
Sample question: What proportion of patients undergoing the surgical procedure are smokers?	**Sample question:** Is there a relationship between smoking and poor functional outcomes after a specific spine surgery?

Table 6-4   Differences between univariate and bivariate data analyses.

Parametric versus nonparametric tests

When making comparisons or measuring associations between two variables, the first decision that needs to be made before choosing the specific test is what type of data you will be collecting. Many statistical tests are based upon the assumption that the data are sampled from a normal distribution (ie, bell-shaped curve distribution also known as a Gaussian distribution). These tests, such as the two-sample t test for continuous data, are referred to as parametric tests. Tests that do not make assumptions about the population distribution (usually because the data is not normally distributed) are referred to as nonparametric tests (**Table 6-5**). The chi-square test and Fisher exact test are common examples and are used for categorical variables. Other examples include the Wilcoxon rank sum test, Mann-Whitney test, and Kruskal-Wallis tests. These nonparametric tests rank the outcome variable from low to high, and then analyze the ranks to determine if the groups being compared are from the same population. You should definitely choose a parametric test if you are sure that your data are sampled from a population with a normal distribution (at least approximately normal). You should select a nonparametric test in the following situations:

• The outcome is a rank or a score, and the population is clearly not normally distributed, such as in disease severity score rankings or the Visual Analogue Score for pain.
• The data are measurements, and you are confident that the population is non-normally distributed (if the data are not sampled from a normal distribution, you should consider whether the values can be transformed and distributed normally).
• When evaluating categorical variables (nominal or ordinal).

Type of data				
Objective	**Parametric test**	**Non-parametric test**	**Dichotomous (two possible outcomes)**	**Survival time**
Descriptive, one group	Mean, SD	Median, IQR	Proportion (rate)	Kaplan Meier survival curve
Compare two unpaired groups	Unpaired *t* test	Mann-Whitney test	Chi-square test (Fisher exact test for small cell sizes)	Log-rank test or Mantel-Haenszel
Compare two paired groups	Paired *t* test	Wilcoxon test	McNemar test	Conditional proportional hazards regression
Compare three or more unmatched groups	One-way analysis of variance (ANOVA)	Kruskal-Wallis test	Chi-square test	Cox proportional hazards regression
Compare three or more matched groups	Repeated-measures ANOVA	Friedman test	Cochrane Q	Conditional proportional hazards regression
Quantify association between two variables	Pearson correlation	Spearman correlation	Chi-square test (Fisher exact test for small cell sizes)	
Predict value from another measured variable	Simple linear regression	Nonparametric regression	Simple logistic regression	Cox proportional hazards regression
Predict value from several measured variables	Multiple linear regression		Multiple logistic regression	Cox proportional hazards regression

Table 6-5   Selecting the appropriate test based on the study's objectives [2].

How do you determine if a distribution is normal?
It is not always easy to know if a sample comes from a normal distribution. If hundreds of data points are collected, then you can inspect the distribution of the data and it will be fairly obvious whether the distribution is approximately bell shaped. A formal statistical test (such as the Kolmogorov-Smirnoff test, which is not discussed in this book) can be used to determine whether the distribution of the data differs significantly from a normal distribution. With only a few data points, it is difficult to tell whether the data are normal by inspection, and the formal test has little power to discriminate between normal and non-normal distributions.

Does it matter whether you choose a parametric or nonparametric test?
The answer depends on the sample size. One rule of thumb is that unless the population distribution is obviously non-normally distributed, you are probably safe choosing a parametric test when there are at least 20 to 30 data points in each group. Parametric tests are more robust, ie, they have greater power to detect differences relative to sample size. With nonparametric tests, the probability of rejecting the null hypothesis is lower.

What happens if you use the wrong test?

With large samples, nonparametric tests are only slightly less powerful than parametric tests. Nonparametric tests generally lack statistical power with small samples. Therefore, large data sets generally do not present problems. With a large data set, it is usually easy to tell if the data come from a normal population, but it does not really matter since the nonparametric tests are nearly as powerful and the parametric tests are rarely affected by outliers. Small data sets, however, can present a problem. It is difficult to tell if the data come from a normal distribution, which is important. With small data sets, nonparametric tests are not as powerful, while parametric tests are affected by outliers.

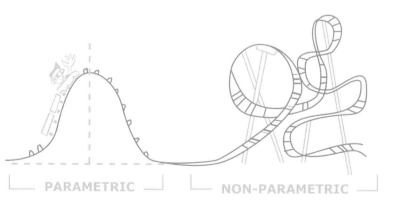

PARAMETRIC   NON-PARAMETRIC

Choosing the correct test for bivariate analyses

The most common statistical tests used for categorical variables are the chi-square test and Fisher exact test. The chi-square test compares the tallies or counts of categorical responses between two or more independent groups. The chi-square test is typically the test of choice with larger study samples. The usual rule of thumb for deciding whether the chi-square approximation is good enough is that the chi-square test is not suitable when the expected values in any of the cells of a contingency table are below five. For example, a sample of patients undergoing cervical fusion might be divided into smokers and nonsmokers when comparing union to nonunion. We hypothesize that the proportion of smokers is higher among the nonunion outcomes than union outcomes. We also want to test whether any difference of proportions that we observe is significant. The data might look like **Table 6-6**.

	Smoker	Non-smoker	Total
Union	2	7	9
Nonunion	9	3	12
Total	11	10	21

Table 6-6   Hypothetical outcomes comparing union rates between smokers and nonsmokers after cervical fusion.

These data would not be suitable for analysis by a chi-square test because some of the values in **Table 6-6** are below five.

When examining a subject population, continuous outcomes are usually reported as means with SDs for normally distributed data or medians with IQRs for non-normally distributed data. A two-sample *t* test is the most common way to estimate whether the mean value of a normally distributed outcomes measurement is significantly different between two groups of subjects. This test is also known as the Student's *t* test or an independent samples *t* test. Two-sample *t* tests are typically used when the outcome is continuous and when the treatment or risk factor (also known as an explanatory variable) is dichotomous. For example, this test would be used to assess whether the mean score of the Oswestry low back pain disability questionnaire is significantly different between patients who have lumbar surgery compared with those who are managed conservatively.

Other tests used when evaluating the association between continuous variables are linear regression and correlation. You should calculate the correlation if you measured both X and Y in each subject and wish to quantify how well they are associated. Select the Pearson (parametric) correlation coefficient if you can assume that both X and Y are sampled from normal populations. Otherwise choose the Spearman rank nonparametric correlation coefficient. Linear regression should be used only if one of the variables (X) is likely to precede or cause the other variable (Y). Definitely choose linear regression if the X variable is changing or being manipulated (eg, the effect of two treatment methods on an outcome).

Multivariate analysis and regression
Regression refers to a set of techniques for modeling and analyzing several variables when the focus is on the relationship between a dependent variable and one or more independent variables. Regression methods allow for evaluation of multiple explanatory variables. This is a useful tool when there is an uneven distribution of risk factors among comparison groups and you want to control and adjust for them, while trying to estimate the effect of a single factor (eg, treatment A versus treatment B). This allows us to control for these variables, thereby minimizing confounding and subsequent bias in the

results (chapter 8: Bias reduction). Regression is also capable of testing interactions between variables, such as assessing statistical effect modification (chapter 9.2: Heterogeneity of treatment effects). When more than a few variables or strata are formed for a stratified analysis, or when more than a few potential confounding factors need to be adjusted, multiple regression can be used. Since a two-sample *t* test, chi-square test, or Fisher exact test can only be used to assess the significance of the difference between the values of two independent groups, regression methods allow for more flexibility.

Linear regression can be used to assess the association or difference between two groups, while controlling for other factors that may be potential confounders (chapter 8: Bias reduction) when the outcome of interest is a continuous variable. In a simple, single predictor variable linear regression or multiple linear regression, the size of the coefficient for each indepen-

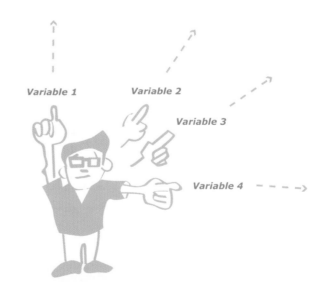

Variable 1　　Variable 2

Variable 3

Variable 4

dent variable gives you the size of the effect that variable is having on your dependent variable. The sign on the coefficient (positive or negative) gives you the direction of the effect. In linear regression with a single independent variable, the coefficient tells you how much the dependent variable is expected to increase (if the coefficient is positive) or decrease (if the coefficient is negative) when that independent variable increases by one. In linear regression with multiple independent variables, the coefficient tells you how much the dependent variable is expected to increase when that independent variable increases by one, while holding all the other independent variables constant. Remember to keep in mind the units in which your variables are measured. Similarly, an ANOVA can be used to compare mean values of three or more independent groups. A similar method known as analysis of covariance (ANCOVA) also allows for inclusion of other risk factors to minimize confounding bias.

There are other types of regression. For dichotomous outcomes, the most common regression technique is logistic regression. Logistic regression is a useful way of describing the relationship between one or more independent variables (eg, age, gender) and a binary response variable expressed as a probability, which has only two values, such as presence or absence of a postoperative complication. The effect measure produced by logistic regression is an odds ratio, which is simply a ratio of odds. In general, they refer to the ratio of the odds of an event occurring in the exposed group versus the unexposed group. Odds ratios can help determine how strongly a given variable may be associated with the outcome of interest compared with other variables. Odds ratios are simply a different way of expressing this association than relative risk since they compare the odds rather than the risk of an event. However, they are sometimes close to each other, such as when the outcome of interest is rare. Therefore, logistic regression is

recommended primarily for uncommon outcomes. Otherwise, the odds ratio will overestimate the relative risk comparing one treatment with another or exposed with unexposed [3]. Other regression methods, such as Cox regression and negative binomial regression, also provide an effect estimate while allowing you to control for other factors. These regressions can produce relative risks instead of odds ratios as effect estimates (in Cox regression they are called hazard ratios). Relative risks are more intuitive than odds ratios, especially when the binary outcome you are assessing is common (ie, occurs more than 10% of the time).

Despite the flexibility and power of regression techniques, they should always be used with caution. You should always plan your study to start with examining univariate and bivariate analyses, first so that you understand your outcome distribution, the potential factors related to outcome, and the potential factors related to each other.

When considering the strength of the effect estimate (RR or OR) from a regression model, the *P* value is less important than the confidence interval. Extremely wide confidence intervals indicate wide variability and the estimate may not be stable. Results for which estimates are surrounded by wide confidence intervals should be interpreted with caution even when associations are statistically significant.

6.6   SMART analysis plan checklist

This chapter has covered a lot of material yet hardly scratches the surface of theories and methods in biostatistics. Although this book focuses on the SMART planning of a clinical study, you must also understand some of the basic principles of study execution and analysis since the proper planning of these tasks ensures a quality execution.

The following checklist should be considered when planning your analysis and can be used when developing your study protocol.

☑ A restatement of your study questions and study design.

☑ A firm understanding of your measurement variables used to answer your study questions.

☑ Power and sample size calculation based on your primary objectives.

☑ A plan for developing data collection forms and a database that allows you to execute your analysis plan seamlessly after finishing your data collection efforts.

☑ An analysis plan for each study question or objective. This begins first with how to handle the descriptive data and then a specific analytical plan for each question if you are making treatment comparisons or assessing risk factor associations.

6.7   Summary

•   For a study to have a reasonable chance of answering its study questions there must be enough subjects. Perform a sample size calculation. Once the sample size has been determined, you need to consider whether a sample of this size is even possible.

•   It is critical that you design a database that will generate as clean of a data set as possible with accurate variables and the fewest missing data points as possible, before starting the analysis.

•   Measurements are usually categorical or continuous. Most analyses are divided into descriptive and analytical statistics and should be clearly described in the methods section of your study. The purpose of analytical statistics is to report the effects of treatment and risk factors for specific outcomes. These rely on the testing of statistical hypotheses. There should be an analytical test for each objective.

•   In order to better understand your data, bivariate analyses should be performed prior to more sophisticated methods of regression.

•   When making comparisons or measuring associations between two variables, the first decision that needs to be made before choosing the specific test is to determine the type of data: parametric or nonparametric. Parametric tests are used to assess normally distributed data and nonparametric for non-normally distributed data.

- The most common statistical tests used for categorical variables are the chi-square test and Fisher exact test.

- The most common test for assessing the difference between two continuous measures is the two-sample t test. Other tests used when evaluating the association between continuous variables are linear regression and correlation.

- Two-sample t tests, chi-square tests, or Fisher exact tests can only be used to assess the significance of the difference between the values of two independent groups, while regression methods allow more flexibility. Linear regression can be used to assess the association or difference between two groups, while controlling for other factors that may be potential confounders when the outcome of interest is a continuous variable.

- Logistic regression is a useful way of describing the relationship between one or more independent variables and a binary response variable, expressed as a probability. The effect measure produced is an odds ratio. Other regression techniques can produce relative risks instead of odds ratios as effect estimates.

- Statistical analyses and associated tests can become far more complex when dealing with non-normally distributed data, paired-data, correlated data, as well as other issues, such as repeated measurements. These are beyond the scope of this book but can be learned in statistical textbooks or by seeking the consultation of a biostatistician or epidemiologist.

6.8   References

1. Greenough CG, Fraser RD (1992) *Assessment of outcome in patients with low-back pain.* Spine; 17(1):36–41.
2. Motulsky H (1995) Intuitive Biostatistics. *New York: Oxford University Press Inc.*
3. Zhang J, Yu KF (1998) What's the relative risk? A method of correcting the odds ratio in cohort studies of common outcomes. *JAMA;* 280(19):1690–1691.

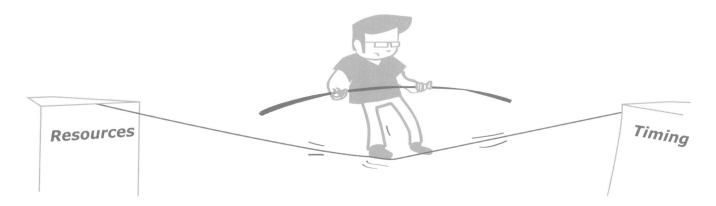

Get your work funded.
It's a team effort.
Plan your timeline.

7 Resources and Timing

7.1 Introduction

The goal of this book is to assist you in planning future clinical research studies, so that you will work smarter and not harder. Overseeing your research on your own without the collaboration of other experts can be an almost impossible undertaking. With a SMART planning approach to resources and timing, you can advance your clinical and academic career without compromising clinical care.

At this point, your study questions, study design, measurements, and analysis plan have been defined and presumably documented in your study protocol. Now that you know what you want to do, how do you go about doing it?

- Who is going to oversee the study operations?
- Who is actually going to collect the data? Do you need to hire someone?
- Who is going to query the data, clean it, and manage the database?
- Who is going to perform the data analyses?
- How are these people going to be supported? Where do those funds come from?
- How long will it take to get institutional review board (IRB) approval before you can begin data collection?
- How long will it take to complete the study?

All these questions need to be addressed before the study can begin.

7.2   Building your team and a network of collaborators

Study logistics is often the least glamorous but necessary part of the study.

This chapter briefly discusses the following issues:

- Building your team and a network of collaborators
- Can you proceed without funding? What funding options do you have?
- What is the cost of data collection and study operations?
- Are there indirect costs?
- Timing and frequency of measurement and length of follow-up

A discussion of the logistics related to multi-site clinical trials is beyond the scope of this book. Although many of these principles also apply to multi-site clinical trials, the amount of support and funding required is significantly greater in those larger studies.

Getting started is often the hardest part of research. Whenever possible, it is advisable to partner with a senior mentor who has clinical research experience in your area of interest. Such a partner is likely to already have a network of collaborators, and may be able to support you in obtaining the necessary resources.

If you are starting from scratch and do not have substantial experience in research, then building a team and a network of collaborators can be challenging. You have to identify the needs of the study and figure out how to fulfill them. At a minimum, all studies require resources for adequate planning, data collection and organization, data analysis, and manuscript preparation. A number of people can assist in these tasks, though identifying collaborators with experience in all these areas is highly recommended. For example, data collection and organization can be done by you the principal investigator, a study coordinator/research assistant, a clinical assistant, or a trainee (eg, fellow, resident, or student). A SMART approach is to delegate or outsource this work to available personnel if there is sufficient funding. However, as the principal investigator, you should maintain oversight regardless of your team's level of expertise since you are ultimately responsible for the success or failure of the study.

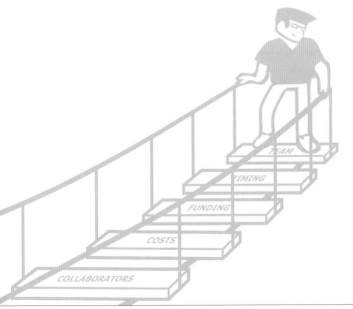

Setting up a user-friendly database with such programs as Excel or Access may require additional assistance. There are specific procedures that should be followed when setting up a database that is conducive for later analysis (chapter 6: Analysis). You may be able to identify internal staff with experience in database development or outsource this task if the funding is available. You will also want someone to regularly manage your data to ensure that it is of the highest quality and functionality.

Data analysis requires an individual familiar with biostatistics. Personnel performing this task should have a thorough understanding of statistical methods and the tools available to perform them. If there is uncertainty, then consultation with a statistician or someone familiar with statistical analysis in clinical research is advisable.

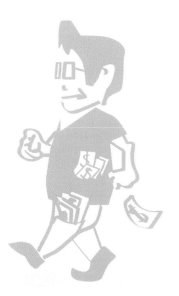

7.3   Can you proceed without funding? What funding options do you have?

Funding requirements can vary based on the study design. Retrospective studies, in general, require far less funding than prospective studies. For a retrospective study, presumably all the data of interest have already been logged in the medical record, and it is just a matter of chart review and data organization. This can often be done in your own time without the burden of collecting data in real time. This can be done by a student, resident, fellow, nurse, physician's assistant, or yourself. Funding requirements for data harvesting may vary from a full-time research assistant to no funding at all if the work is all done by you the principal investigator. For a retrospective study, the activities and team roles that may require funding include:

- Assistance with study design and research methodology
- Sample size calculations
- Study coordinator with experience reviewing medical records and local IRB requirements (if necessary)
- Personnel to collect and/or abstract data, as well as make sure that data quality is not compromised (this may be your study coordinator or a resident)
- Data entry and secure database development
- Statistical analysis

For a prospective study, much more extensive planning is necessary and funding is more frequently required. A busy clinical schedule may preclude you the principal investigator from being able to perform much of the study yourself. Thus, assistance is generally advisable. Unlike retrospective studies, data are collected in real time for prospective studies, and assistance is often required. Specific activities and team roles that may require funding for a prospective study include:

- Assistance with study design, research methodology, and the operations of prospective data collection efforts
- Sample size calculations
- Study coordinator with experience in project management, recruitment, prospective data collection efforts, and IRB requirements (generally advisable)
- A highly trained person to interview subjects (if applicable) and to collect and/or abstract data (this may be your study coordinator)
- Development of a secure database
- Data entry and database management
- Measurement of outcomes, such as clinical outcomes scores or radiographic outcomes
- Statistical analysis
- Manuscript preparation (if assistance needed)

It is recommended that statistical analysis be done by an individual with the appropriate education and training. Statistical analysis can range from simple analytical tests (t test, chi-square test) to complex multivariate regression analyses. While simple tests can often be performed by anyone who has a rudimentary understanding of them, it is advisable that the complex analyses be performed by an individual with formal education and training in statistical analysis. Additional funding may be required for the data analysis (chapter 6: Analysis).

7.4   Possible funding sources

Numerous funding sources exist to support research efforts. When applying for grant funding, it is important to align the parameters of your study to the parameters of the grant and priorities of the granting agency. Whereas some grants are limited by the total funding amount, others may require a prospective nature of data harvest, while some may require the study of a specific area of research. One should also be particularly mindful of other possible restrictions and obligations that may accompany funding. Examples of funding sources include:

- Governmental funding
  - National Institute of Health (www.nih.gov)
  - Veteran Health Administration (www.va.gov)
- Professional societies
  - AOSpine (www.aospine.org)
  - North American Spine Society (www.spine.org)
  - Cervical Spine Research Society (www.csrs.og)
  - Scoliosis Research Society (www.srs.org)
  - Orthopedic Research and Education Foundation (www.oref.org)
- Institutional
- Departmental
- Industry
- Self-funding (Depending on the size of the study or task, the availability or lack of funding, and the importance of the project, never rule out the possibility of self-funding as an option for advancing your career.)

Applications for funding from the government or professional societies require a detailed budget. Thus, accounting for all direct and indirect costs a priori is essential. In addition, these funding sources generally require a midterm progress report and a final report, whereas departmental funding may not.

7.5 What is the cost of data collection and study operations?

In addition to hiring personnel to collect the data, you must also be mindful of the cost of the study operations and data management. Always consider administrative costs, such as paper, technology, postage, telephone calls, and other indirect costs. These often apply to a university or a medical center. When applying for a grant or funding, the hosting institution can often charge a certain amount of overhead or indirect costs. These costs are meant to support university infrastructure where the research is conducted. Indirect costs vary per institution. Conversely, sponsors can limit what percentage of funding awarded is used toward indirect costs.

Furthermore, some clinical measurements may have proprietary restrictions and incur costs associated with their use. If radiographic outcomes are to be used outside the normal postoperative routine, then these studies may need to be funded. For example, if you wish to obtain a CT scan 1 year after fusion in all patients, funding may be needed to support these studies. While a CT scan to assess for pseudarthrosis in a symptomatic patient is within the routine standard of care, a CT scan to assess for fusion in an asymptomatic patient for research purposes may require additional funding. In addition, you should consider creating an appropriate database with de-identified data that is compliant with local or multi-site IRB requirements including appropriate security and back-up measures. There is also time and cost associated with regular data management including data entry, quality assurance checks, and querying of missing and nonsensical data.

7.6 Timing

There are several aspects to timing. First, it is directly related to the discussion on resources and funding. When applying for funding through granting agencies, it is essential to plan the timeline. Can this study be completed during the allotted time with the funding that you are applying for? A sample timeline is presented in **Table 7-1** for a prospective study seeking 1-year follow-up data on patients enrolled.

As noted in **Table 7-1**, the timeline can be affected by numerous factors that need to be considered. You the principal investigator should have a sense of how frequently patients are treated. Sometimes the timeline can be affected by the frequency of disease observation, such as trauma or tumor. The amount of time needed to recruit a sufficient number of patients can vary widely, and this has an obvious effect on the length of the study.

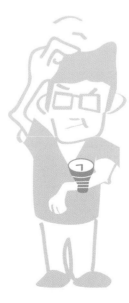

Project milestones	Year 1		Year 2				Year 3				Year 4	
	Q3	Q4	Q1	Q2	Q3	Q4	Q1	Q2	Q3	Q4	Q1	Q2
Planning/IRB approval/ secure funding	X	X										
Enrollment of patients into the study			X	X	X	X						
Prospectively record perioperative data and 6-week follow-up				X	X	X	X					
Prospectively record 6-month to 1-year follow-up data (clinical and radiographic outcomes)						X	X	X	X	X	X	
Analysis of data; preliminary preparation of abstract and manuscript									X	X		
Presentation of data; preparation of manuscript											X	X
Prepare final report (abstract and manuscript)												X

Table 7-1   Sample study timeline. Q1, Q2, Q3, and Q4 indicate the four quarters of the year.

The timeline of a retrospective study differs greatly from a prospective study. As mentioned before, in a retrospective study, all the data are presumably recorded and it is simply a matter of reviewing the medical record, harvesting the data, and analyzing it. Nonetheless, you still need to plan time to have these things done. You need to consider how much time it takes for each of these tasks and set timelines for completing them.

In a prospective study, theoretically you should design your study with planned follow-up time points and then subsequently determine costs afterward. However, the reality is that funding resources may limit the frequency and length of follow-up. You may not be able to obtain data points every 3 months and may be limited to 1- or 2-year follow-ups depending on how you would like to examine the intervention. In addition, some prospective studies may consider paying subjects for attending follow-up appointments as an incentive. Since this is an additional cost, a greater number of follow-ups requiring subject participation may increase cost in addition to other study duties such as project management, data entry, and data management. This all ties back into your overall timeline.

Although timing is a latter component of the SMART approach, you should be mindful of timing throughout all aspects of the study. When crafting the study question, or considering the measurements or analysis, parallel considerations of resources and timing are necessary to execute a study efficiently. Often timing may be the rate-limiting step, and these limitations may direct you toward a different strategy.

7.7   Summary

- When considering resources and timing of a study, planning and documentation of your plan is paramount. While retrospective chart review studies can be done with less preparation and planning, a prospective study requires detailed planning before the first patient is enrolled.

- In parallel with the planning of the study, one should consider resource and timing requirements. Planning costs can include employing an epidemiologist or study methodologist for study design, statistician or data analyst, research coordinator, and database manager. Study execution costs may include: clinical outcome measurements, performance and interpretation of radiographic studies, and personnel to harvest and organize data in real time and possibly compensation for participant time and participation. Post-study costs can include a biostatistician for data analysis, as well as personnel assistance for manuscript preparation, formatting, and presentation. Indirect costs may need to be accounted for and are institution-dependent.

- When your study is successfully funded, you must be aware of the requirements and obligations to the study sponsor.

- Planning of the study design, resources, and timing, though tedious and cumbersome, is essential to ensure a smooth execution of the study with minimal changes throughout the process. As with other aspects of the study discussed in previous chapters, all these things should be documented in your study protocol.

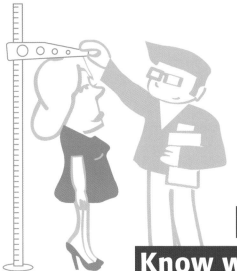

Reduce the potential for bias.
Know what kind of bias occurs when.
Double blind against bias.

8   Bias reduction:
how to avoid spurious conclusions

8.1   Introduction

All studies have the potential for bias, even randomized controlled trials (RCTs). The overall quality of many published studies is poor, making it difficult to draw evidence-based conclusions. This is most frequently attributed to how much (or how little) investigators have taken bias into consideration and designed studies to avoid bias, whether in an RCT or a case series.

The credibility and validity of your study rests in large part with what actions you take to reduce the potential for bias. Part of your SMART plan needs to include consideration of the types of bias and explicit steps to minimize their influence on the quality of your results and the conclusions that can be drawn from them. Consultation with those experienced in clinical study methodology will be helpful here as well.

In some ways, this is the most important chapter in this book. It outlines the primary sources of bias in studies and makes suggestions for study design and analyses that minimize bias. An understanding of the common sources of study bias also facilitates your critical appraisal of other published studies.

What is bias and how do we avoid it?

The extent to which an individual can draw conclusions about the effects of an exposure (ie, how much one can infer that a cause and effect relationship exists between the exposure and the outcomes) depends on whether the data and results of a study are valid. This is often referred to as internal validity, which is directly related to how much a study is free from bias.

An exposure is a potential causal characteristic and can refer to a treatment (eg, surgery, drugs), a behavior (eg, smoking), a trait (eg, sex) or, in the simplest sense, anything one may be exposed to (eg, airborne illness). An exposure is sometimes referred to in research as the "independent variable" since it is the factor being varied or manipulated in a study and which determines the change in the dependent variable (ie, outcomes).

Bias is a systematic error or deviation from the truth. It results in either an overestimate or an underestimate of the true effect of an exposure. Said another way, bias is a lack of internal validity or an incorrect or distorted assessment of the association between an exposure and an effect in a target population.

The degree to which one can place confidence in the results of a study depends greatly on whether biases have been accounted for and the necessary steps have been taken to diminish the impact of biases.

Bias can be introduced into a study in a number of ways and each stage of the trial process is prone to a specific type of bias (**Fig 8-1**). Some of the most common and discernible causes of bias are summarized in **Table 8-1**. They include:

- Selection bias—biased assignment to comparison groups
- Attrition bias—biased occurrence and management of loss to follow-up and deviations from protocol
- Performance bias—biased difference in delivery of care and preferential provision of additional care (other than the treatment of interest)
- Measurement/detection bias—biased outcome assessment or classification
- Reporting bias—biased reporting of significant or favorable results

As you will see, mitigating the effects of bias depends greatly on the adequacy of the study design and the degree of control exercised in gathering data.

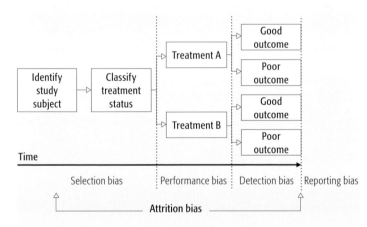

Fig 8-1 Areas of potential bias within the study architecture.

Bias	When it occurs	Effects	Ways to minimize
Selection	Patient selection	• False acceptance or rejection of hypothesis • Distorts effect size • Creates confounding • Nonrepresentative sample	• Random allocation • Allocation concealment • In nonrandomized studies, identify a wide range of prognostic factors and control for them statistically
Attrition	Any phase	• False acceptance or rejection of hypothesis • Distorts effect size • Creates confounding • Nonrepresentative sample	• Intention-to-treat (ITT) analysis • Analyze study "completers" versus "drop-outs" • Sensitivity analysis • Implement processes to help retain participants
Performance	Treatment	• False acceptance or rejection of hypothesis • Distorts effect size	• Blinding • Stratification • Set up and follow specific study protocols
Measurement/ detection	Outcomes measurement	• False acceptance or rejection of hypothesis • Distorts effect size • Misclassification of outcomes	• Independent assessment • Set up and follow specific study protocols • Use valid and reliable measurement instruments • Periodic assessment of measurement process
Reporting	Publication process	• False acceptance or rejection of hypothesis • Distorts effect size	• Provide complete data for all pre-specified outcomes

Table 8-1   Summary table of types of bias and suggestions for minimizing them.

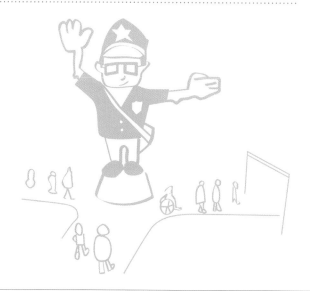

8.2   Selection bias

☞ **Selection bias occurs when individuals are preferentially assigned to treatment or control groups, resulting in systematic differences between the groups that influence prognosis or responsiveness to treatment.**

Selection bias usually exists due to a flaw in the sample selection process, whereby a subset of the population of interest is systematically excluded. Some common examples of situations that lead to selection bias include:

- Self-selection or physician-directed selection of treatments: Self-selection occurs when patients' characteristics cause patients to select themselves for a specific treatment group. Similarly, physician-directed selection happens when patients' characteristics lead the physician to choose those patients for a particular treatment. Both cases create abnormal conditions in the group because there are a number of inherent differences that likely exist between those patients who chose a treatment for themselves and those who do not choose that treatment, and between the patients selected by the physician for a particular treatment and those who are not selected for that treatment. Self-selection makes it difficult to determine causation since there are likely other factors affecting the outcome rather than just the treatment alone. Physician-directed selection is prone to bias because decisions about care can be related to condition severity, prognosis, and responsiveness to treatment.

- Convenience sampling: Sometimes referred to as a type of nonprobability sampling, this occurs when individuals are selected because they are readily available and convenient. This sampling technique is fast, inexpensive, and easy. The problem with this method is that such a sample would likely not be representative enough of the entire population. It can lead to an under-representation or an over-representation of particular groups within the population of interest.

- Association of treatment assignments with demographic, clinical, or social characteristics: Often certain patient characteristics, such as disease severity or comorbidity, naturally suggest treatment. When these characteristics that influence treatment choice also influence the patient's prognosis, confounding by indication can result. This is primarily a concern in observational studies since the allocation of treatment is not randomized and the indication for treatment may be related to the risk of future health outcomes. The resulting imbalance in the underlying risk profile between treatment and control groups can generate biased results and may be extremely important to consider in studies of efficacy or safety.

For instance, a prospective cohort study by Ugwonali et al [1] assessed outcomes following brace treatment compared with observation in an idiopathic scoliosis population. Baseline demographics reveal that patients who underwent bracing had a mean Cobb angle of 34.5° compared with 24.6° in those who received observation alone, suggesting that those who got a brace had more severe disease. The best way to prevent confounding by indication is to ensure that patients with the same range of condition severity are included in both treatment groups and that choice of treatment is not based on condition severity.

- Use of historical controls: An historical control group is one that is chosen from a group of patients who were treated in the past. The group treated in the past is used for comparison with subjects being treated currently. The use of historical controls raises concerns about valid comparisons, since they are likely to differ from the current treatment group in their composition, diagnosis, disease severity, determination of outcomes, and/or other important ways that would confound the treatment effect. Furthermore, the issue of "secular trend" in medicine (which refers to the changes that occur over time related to healthcare delivery and advances and/or changes in surgical methods and equipment, etc) could cause distinct differences between the treatment groups and possibly influence outcomes.

☞ **There are various ways that selection bias influences the results of a study. It may result in falsely accepting or rejecting a hypothesis. It may distort the estimate of association between risk factor and disease or between treatment and outcome.**

Selection bias can create confounding through unequal distribution of patients with a specific attribute (eg, more serious condition) between study arms. It can also result in patients in the sample being unrepresentative of the population of interest, limiting the applicability or generalizability of the study.

The best ways to limit or eliminate the effects of selection bias is to use randomization and allocation concealment when creating study groups. Randomization ensures that potential confounding factors, known or unknown, are evenly distributed among the study groups. This creates two groups with similar characteristics, minimizing any bias that might affect the relationship between the intervention and the outcome of interest. Allocation concealment is a method used to prevent participants, investigators, and others involved in the research study from learning about group assignments prior to the start of the study. This inhibits healthcare providers from (even un-knowingly) influencing enrollment or the selection of participating subjects and prevents patients from choosing the intervention they desire. The effects of an intervention tend to be overestimated without allocation concealment. In fact, trials with inadequate allocation concealment have been shown to yield estimates of treatment effect up to 40% larger than trials using adequate allocation concealment [2, 3]. Therefore, a large treatment effect from a randomized trial without adequate allocation concealment might simply reflect biased allocation [4]. In nonrandomized studies, when known baseline prognostic factors are collected, one can reduce the effect of selection bias during the analysis phase by using statistical methods, such as stratification and multivariate regression.

What is confounding?

☞ **Confounding is often referred to as a mixing of effects, wherein the effects of an extraneous factor (confounder) blend in with the effects of the exposure of interest on a given outcome. The result is a falsification of the true relationship.**

A confounding variable causes a problem because it is empirically related to both the exposure and the outcome and may compete with the exposure of interest (eg, treatment) in explaining the outcome of a study. The existence of confounding variables in studies make it difficult to establish a clear causal link between treatment and outcome unless appropriate methods are used to adjust for the effect of the confounders. If the effect of the confounders can be removed, one can obtain a more appropriate estimate of the true association that is due to the exposure. General characteristics of confounders include the following:

Predictive of the outcome

A confounding factor is predictive of the outcome even in the absence of the exposure (**Fig 8-2**). A confounding factor is associated with the outcome and not the result of the exposure or the outcome. Many confounding factors are proxies for variables that are complex and difficult to measure.

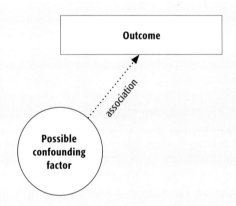

Fig 8-2   Confounding factors are predictive of the outcome.

For example, elderly people tend to heal more slowly compared with younger people, making them more prone to develop complications like nonunion or delayed union after a bone fracture. Age is therefore associated with a greater risk of these complications regardless of the exposure (treatment) used.

Associated with the exposure

A confounding factor is also associated with the exposure being studied, but is not a proxy or surrogate for the exposure (**Fig 8-3**). In clinical trials, confounding is often a result of unequal distribution of the potential confounding factors between treatment groups.

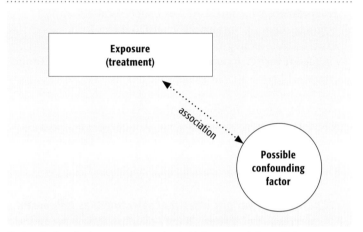

Fig 8-3   Confounding factors are also associated with the exposure being studied.

A situation that contains both **Fig 8-2** and **Fig 8-3** sets the stage for potential confounding (**Fig 8-4**).

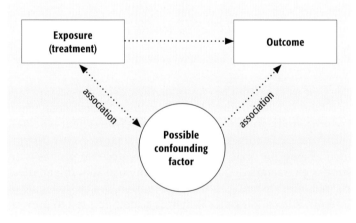

Fig 8-4   A confounding factor that is both predictive of the outcome and associated with the exposure.

Not an intermediate between the exposure and outcome
A confounding factor cannot be an intermediate between the exposure and outcome (**Fig 8-5**). For example, the relationship between sex and osteoporotic vertebral fractures may be explained by measuring bone mineral density. Bone mass is not a confounder because it may be a causal link between sex and osteoporotic vertebral fractures.

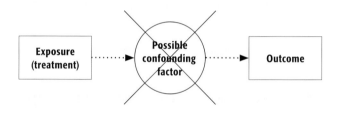

Fig 8-5   Confounding factors cannot be intermediates between the exposure and outcome.

How does confounding influence results?

Let us imagine that we want to know if treating index osteoporotic vertebral fractures with vertebroplasty increased the risk of subsequent vertebral fractures. We evaluate 400 patients with index vertebral fractures, of whom 200 received vertebroplasty, and 200 did not. After 2 years, we indentify 45 subsequent fractures with the hypothetical distribution in **Table 8-2**.

Vertebroplasty	Conservative care	Risk ratio (95% confidence interval)
30/200 (15%)	15/200 (7.5%)	2.0 (1.1–3.6)

Table 8-2   Hypothetical distribution of subsequent vertebral fractures after treating index osteoporotic vertebral fractures.

At first glance, it looks like those who received vertebroplasty were at a much higher risk (twice the risk) compared with those who did not. This is called a crude estimate of the association. However, it is important to investigate whether other reasons could account for this difference. In particular, other variables that may influence the risk of subsequent vertebral fractures should be evaluated, such as age, weight, and smoking status. **Table 8-3** describes these variables at the time of the incident fracture. Note that age and weight are similar between groups. However, the difference in the proportion of patients who smoke is dramatically different, with 55% in the vertebroplasty group compared with only 8% in the conservative care group.

	Vertebroplasty N = 200	Conservative care N = 200
Age (years), mean ± SD	78.2 ± 4.1	79.0 ± 5.2
Weight (kg), mean ± SD	54.4 ± 2.3	53.9 ± 2.1
Smoking status (n)	110 (55%)	16 (8%)

Table 8-3   Other variables that may influence subsequent vertebral fractures. SD indicates standard deviation.

If we stratify the results by smoking status (**Table 8-4**), we note that the risk of subsequent fractures is similar between treatment groups in each stratum (smoking and nonsmoking), such that the risk ratio is closer to 1 (no effect) compared with the crude results in **Table 8-2** where the risk ratio was 2.

Smoking			Nonsmoking		
Vertebroplasty	Conservative	RR (95% CI)	Vertebroplasty	Conservative	RR (95% CI)
23/110 (21%)	3/16 (19%)	1.1 (0.4– 3.3)	7/90 (8%)	12/184 (7%)	1.2 (0.5– 2.9)

Table 8-4   Stratified results by smoking status. RR indicates risk ratio and CI indicates confidence interval.

Thus, smoking was a confounding factor distorting the true relationship between vertebroplasty and the risk of subsequent vertebral fractures.

Dealing with confounding

The potential for confounding should be considered in the design and implementation of your study. For a nonrandomized study, factors that might be associated with the outcome other than the treatment need to be measured. To some extent, confounding can be accounted for during analysis, assuming that such factors have been measured as part of the study.

Step 1: Measure and report all potential confounders

It is extremely important to quantify and report patient characteristics, since they may be potential confounders. However, patient characteristics are unfortunately often an underreported or misreported set of measurements in spine care studies. Diagnostic features, comorbidities, and any factor that might affect patient outcomes need to be measured and reported for each study group as well. Authors often include a demographic or patient characteristic table at the beginning of their study articles, making it possible to determine at a glance whether the groups are comparable. However, as mentioned previously, these tables are often insufficient and omit pertinent details about the study groups. **Table 8-5** presents a good example of a demographic table that is robust and comprehensive. Any and all of these characteristics, features, and factors may be potential confounders of the relationship between the exposure of interest (eg, a surgical treatment) and the outcome (eg, patient function). Planning for and measuring these attributes goes a long way toward dealing with the role of confounding.

	Surgery n=176 (%)	Rehabilitation n=173(%)
Male	79 (44.9)	93 (53.8)
Female	97 (55.1)	80 (46.2)
Age		
• <30 years	24 (13.6)	20 (11.6)
• 30–39 years	63 (35.8)	67 (38.7)
• 40–49 years	56 (31.8)	66 (38.1)
• ≥50 years	33(18.8)	20 (11.6)
Treatment center		
• A	55 (31.3)	54 (31.2)
• B	28 (15.9)	27 (15.6)
• C	45 (25.6)	43 (24.9)
• D	48 (27.3)	49 (28.3)
Mean duration of back pain in years (range)	8 (1–35)	8 (1–35)
Current smokers	76 (43.2)	74 (42.8)
Litigation	25 (14.2)	21 (12.1)
Currently in paid employment	88 (50.0)	94 (54.3)
Back pain interfered with patient's ability to work	149 (84.7)	149 (86.1)
• Had to give up job	65 (43.6)	67 (45.0)
• Had to change job	19 (12.7)	10 (6.7)
• Had to reduce hours	17 (11.4)	12 (8.0)
• Had to take sick leave	59 (39.6)	69 (46.3)
Comorbid disease*	55 (31.3)	48 (27.7)
Clinical classification		
• Spondylolisthesis	20 (11.4)	18 (10.4)

	Surgery n=176 (%)	Rehabilitation n=173(%)
• Postlaminectomy	14 (8.0)	14 (8.1)
• Chronic low back pain	142 (80.6)	141 (81.5)
Planned surgery type		
• Graft	27 (15.3)	28 (16.2)
• Fusion	149 (84.7)	144 (83.2)
• Missing	0	1 (0.6)
Planned fused level		
• Single level	100 (56.8)	109 (63.0)
• >1 level	70 (39.8)	62 (35.8)
• Missing	6 (3.4)	2 (1.2)
Baseline Oswestry Disability Index†	46.5 (14.6)	44.8 (14.8)
Baseline shuttle walking test in meters†	254 (209)	247 (185)
Baseline SF-36 physical component score†	19.4 (8.8)	20 (9.7)
Baseline SF-36 mental component score†	43.2 (10.9)	44.2 (12.6)
Baseline modified somatic perception questionnaire†	9.0 (6.4)	7.7 (5.7)
Baseline Zung self-rating depression scale†	31.8 (10.4)	31.2 (11.8)
Baseline distress and risk assessment method†		
• Normal	14 (8.0)	14 (8.1)
• At risk	65 (36.9)	85 (49.1)
• Distressed depressive	87 (49.4)	69 (39.9)
• Distressed somatic	9 (5.1)	2 (1.2)
• Missing	1 (0.6)	3 (1.7)

Table 8-5 Baseline patient characteristics and clinical details at trial entry. Adapted from a randomized controlled trial by Fairbank et al [5].
*Any self-reported chronic pulmonary disease, heart disease, stroke, cancer, or diabetes.
†Mean score (SD).

Step 2: Routinely assess the role of confounding factors and adjust for them in your analyses

There are a number of ways of assessing and adjusting for confounding; however, a detailed discussion of this is beyond the scope of this chapter. Briefly, a few examples of how this could be accomplished include:

• During study planning, inclusion could be restricted by specific confounding variables, such as age.
• Several methods of adjusting the effect estimate as part of the analysis can be used. Stratification is one method that can be relatively straightforward and involves looking at the association between the exposure and outcome for each factor category (or stratum) by calculating a stratum-specific estimate.
• Multivariate analysis, a set of statistical methods that allows for adjustment of multiple variables simultaneously via mathematical modeling, can also be used to control for confounding.

Step 3: Report adjusted and crude estimates of association and discuss the study limitations that may be due to confounding and the magnitude of their influence

Regardless of the method used, an adjusted estimate should be obtained that reflects the degree of association between the exposure and disease that remains after the effects of the confounder have been removed. In general, if the adjusted estimate is different from the crude estimate (ie, the association ignoring extraneous factors) by approximately 10% or more, the factor should be considered a confounder and the adjusted estimate used as a more reliable indicator of the effect of the exposure, ie, as an estimate of the effect above and beyond that which is due to the confounders.

In summary, failure to evaluate demographic and baseline clinical factors as potential confounders can bias your study results and lead to erroneous conclusions. Study design must include the measurement and reporting of such factors to allow for comparisons of important characteristics between treatment groups. During analysis, the association between such factors, the outcome, and your exposure of interest must be explored.

In all likelihood, no matter how many variables you adjust for, there will be residual confounding, possibly by factors that are unknown, and therefore, cannot be measured.

8.3 Attrition bias

Attrition bias occurs when there are systematic differences in patients excluded from the study after they have been allocated to treatment groups.

This can happen in two ways. First, when data are collected over two or more points in time, it is common for some participants either to drop out of the study prematurely or to stop the assigned treatment due to medical advice. This is referred to as loss to follow-up since you cannot include these patients' outcomes in the overall results. Second, attrition bias can be introduced into a study through deviations from protocol, such as violation of eligibility criteria and nonadherence to treatment. Patients not adhering to treatment usually differ in respects that are related to prognosis [6].

Attrition bias can potentially change the collective characteristics of the relevant groups and their observed outcomes in ways that adversely affect study results. Those who drop out of the study or who are lost to follow-up may be systematically different from those who remain in the study. For example, if participants who have greater disease severity tend to drop out at a higher rate than those with less disease severity, then a given treatment may appear to be more beneficial than it actually is (in fact, it could be completely ineffective) since the comparison before and after treatment is only in those who finish the study (ie, the healthier study participants). The reverse can also be true. Individuals who feel great and are doing well may drop out of the study because they do not see the need to continue treatment. If only those who complete the study are analyzed, then the results may conclude that the treatment is not effective, when in fact this is not the case. Attrition bias also affects the external validity of the study in that the remaining sample may not be generalizable to the original population that was sampled.

There are a few ways that attrition bias can be detected and corrected.

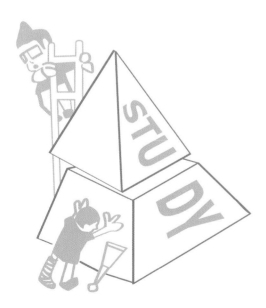

- An intention-to-treat (ITT) analysis can be performed. An ITT analysis is based on the initial treatment intent, not on the treatment eventually administered. Everyone who begins the treatment is considered to be part of the trial, whether he or she finishes or not.
- An analysis can be performed to see if there were differences in various prognostic factors between the study "drop-outs" and "completers".

- A sensitivity analysis can be performed to explore a substantial loss to follow-up. Data are first analyzed including the lost patients as if they were responders to the therapy (best-case scenario) and then as if they were non-responders (worst-case scenario). If the results of both analyses hardly differ, the results can be considered robust, since they are not seriously influenced by those that dropped out. On the other hand, if the analyses differ, then the results are unreliable.

Processes can also be implemented at the outset of a study to help retain patients [7]:

- Fully educating the patients about the demands of the study prior to allocation
- Developing efficient tracking systems to constantly identify the location and status of patients
- Enlisting the support of other healthcare providers who the patients see regularly for follow-up reminders
- Sending out follow-up postcards
- Conducting telephone reminders
- Scheduling follow-up appointment times around patient preferences
- Keeping follow-up interviews brief

8.4   Performance bias

Performance bias occurs when there are systematic differences in the care provided to patients and deviation from the protocol.

This can include differences in care apart from the intervention being evaluated. Some examples include:

- Surgeon experience: Studies from both general and joint surgery literature have demonstrated that a high surgical volume for certain surgical procedures reduces morbidity and improves clinical and economic outcomes [8–14]. Surgeons who perform more procedures have acquired a greater level of skill, familiarity, and precision than a novice surgeon or a surgeon with less patient volume. If patients treated by different surgeons with varying levels of experience are compared, better patient outcomes may be due to the performance of the surgeon and not due to the effectiveness of the procedure itself.

- Unintended interventions or cointerventions: These become a problem when treatments other than the intervention being studied are applied differently to the study and control groups. For example, if patients know they are in the control group, then they may be more likely to use other forms of care. Patients who know they are in the intervention group may experience placebo effects. Treatment-group patients may receive more intensive postoperative care compared with control-group patients. Healthcare providers may treat patients differently according to what group they are in. All these instances introduce bias into the study by creating unequal study conditions that may distort the true effects of the treatment.

- Perioperative care may differ by hospital and institution: This would present a problem in a multicenter study in which the entire study population comprised sample groups treated at different hospitals and institutions. The concern is that differences in perioperative care and hospital procedures might serve to explain differences in outcomes rather than the treatment itself.

- Use of historical controls: As discussed earlier, using a control group who received treatment at an early point in time likely means there are important differences between that group and the current intervention group in regard to composition, diagnosis, disease severity, determination of outcomes, and other important factors that would confound the treatment effect and influence outcomes. The concept of secular trend is important here as well.

The primary effect of performance bias is that any differential treatment may cause a result that is due to the cointervention rather than the active treatment being studied, typically leading to an overestimation of the true treatment effect.

The best way to protect against performance bias is by blinding or masking study participants—ideally both the patients and providers of care—whereby neither the patients nor the providers are aware of which intervention is being allocated. This is referred to as a double-blind experiment. Blinding prevents people from knowing certain information that might lead to conscious or subconscious bias on their part, thus invalidating the results. Another way to limit performance bias would be to stratify the results by surgeon, hospital, etc, in order to ensure that you are comparing apples to apples.

8.5 Measurement or detection bias

Measurement or detection bias occurs when there are systematic differences in outcomes assessment among groups being compared, ie, the accuracy of information collected about or from study participants is not equal between treatment and control groups.

Some examples include:

- Assessor bias: This occurs when an investigator's knowledge about patient assignment influences the outcomes assessment. For instance, nonblinded assessors may provide different measurements and interpretations of borderline x-ray findings or may offer differential encouragement while conducting and recording the results of performance tests.

- Response bias: This occurs when patients either consciously or subconsciously answer questions in a way that they think the investigator wants them to answer. This is most relevant during survey sampling, such as when measuring patient satisfaction. For example, the wording of a question may be loaded in some way to unduly favor one response over another, such as offering only one option for satisfied and two for dissatisfied ("dissatisfied" and "very dissatisfied").

- Recall bias: This occurs in retrospective studies when there are differences in accuracy or completeness of recall of past events or exposures between treatment and control patients, which are not independent of outcome/disease status. For example, there is a tendency for diseased people (or their relatives) to recall past exposures more efficiently than healthy people.

- Faulty instrument or measurement technique: This occurs when a measurement instrument or outcome questionnaire is used that has not been validated or shown to be reliable in the population being studied, which can lead to inappropriate inferences. Using tests and instruments that are valid and reliable to measure outcomes is a crucial component of research quality. An example of a good measurement instrument for use in spine populations is the Oswestry low back pain disability questionnaire. This measure has been shown by numerous studies to be a valid, reliable, and responsive measurement of low back pain in patients with a wide range of spinal disorders [15, 16]. In regard to technique, a faulty measuring process may include inappropriate physical environment, procedural mistakes, and a lack of understanding of the measurement process.

Measurement/detection bias does affect the outcomes of a study since a phenomenon is more or less likely to be observed and reported for a particular set of study participants. It can also lead to misclassification of the exposure or intervention, covariates, or outcomes because of variable definitions and timings.

In order to limit measurement/detection bias, researchers must ensure that similar strategies are used to detect and measure outcomes in all populations being studied. Specification of such factors in the study protocol as part of the study planning is important. Periodic assessment of measurement processes, improving the system of measurements in consultation with an expert, or simply conducting an audit of the measuring process in light of new facts and advancements are all ways to limit measurement/detection bias. As previously discussed, blinding of outcome assessors and independent assessment by someone not vested in the study are key methods for maintaining the accuracy of your results. The use of valid and reliable measurement instruments is critical.

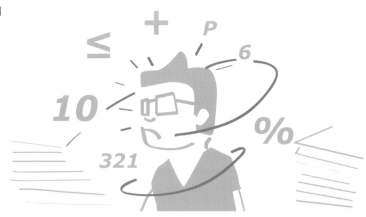

8.6   Reporting bias

Reporting bias occurs when there are systematic differences between reported and unreported findings within a study that are dependent on the nature and direction of the results.

- Differential reporting of outcomes or harms: This refers to the tendency to under-report unexpected or undesirable results, attributing them to sampling or measurement error, while being more trusting of expected or desirable results, though these may be subject to the same source of error.

- Incomplete reporting of study outcomes: This occurs when a study with multiple outcomes reports only those results that were significant and omits insignificant or unfavorable results.

- Funding and author conflict of interest: There is always the potential for bias if the study receives funding from a party with a monetary and proprietary investment in the study outcomes and if the authors have a financial conflict of interest. This influence may lead to the differential reporting of outcomes. For example, Okike et al [17] investigated the association between types of declared conflicts of interest and reported study outcomes in orthopedic research. They found that individuals with a conflict of interest related to royalties, stock options, or consulting and employee status were significantly more likely to describe positive findings.

In other words, a treatment may be considered to be of more value than it merits, depriving patients of more effective or cheaper alternatives, while the suppression of nonsignificant findings could lead to the use of a harmful intervention.

The most immediate effect of reporting bias is that it leads to an overestimation of efficacy and an underestimation of safety risks regarding a given intervention.

In order to limit the effects of reporting bias, complete data should be provided for all prespecified trial outcomes, independent of their results. If this is not the case, try contacting authors for a list of unreported outcomes since this is usually feasible and may have the potential to identify important omissions from publications. Also, it is good practice to search for and include trials in both the published and unpublished literature since this may provide a broader evidence base. Conflicts of interest must be recognized and identified, then managed, reduced, or eliminated. For handling individual investigator conflicts of interest, disclosure and oversight of the research by an independent board is the most common management strategy. However, substantial variability among academic institutions and peer-reviewed journals in their policies governing financial conflicts have been reported [18–22].

8.7   Summary

- Treatment effects may be real, may occur by chance (sampling error), or may be related to other factors, such as bias.

- Bias and confounding are types of error that must be managed in patient selection, data collection, analysis, and data interpretation. These major threats to the internal validity of a study should always be considered as alternative explanations in the interpretation.

- One goal of any good research study should be to minimize bias. In order to limit misinterpretation and misuse of data, clinical investigators and consumers of clinical research should strive to comprehend the residual effects of bias.

8.8 References

1. Ugwonali OF, Lomas G, Choe JC, et al (2004) Effect of bracing on the quality of life of adolescents with idiopathic scoliosis. *Spine J;* 4(3): 254–260.

2. Schulz KF, Chalmers I, Hayes RJ, et al (1995) Empirical evidence of bias. *Dimensions of methodological quality associated with estimates of treatment effects in controlled trials. JAMA;* 273(5):408–412.

3. Schulz KF, Grimes DA (2002) Allocation concealment in randomised trials: defending against deciphering. *Lancet;* 359(9306):614–618.

4. Viera AJ, Bangdiwala SI (2007) Eliminating bias in randomized controlled trials: importance of allocation concealment and masking. *Fam Med;* 39(2):132–137.

5. Fairbank J, Frost H, Wilson-MacDonald J, et al (2005) Randomised controlled trial to compare surgical stabilisation of the lumbar spine with an intensive rehabilitation programme for patients with chronic low back pain: the MRC spine stabilisation trial. *BMJ;* 330(7502):1233.

6. Coronary Drug Project Research Group (1980) Influence of adherence to treatment and response of cholesterol on mortality in the coronary drug project. *N Engl J Med;* 303(18):1038–1041.

7. Sprague S, Leece P, Bhandari M, et al (2003) Limiting loss to follow-up in a multicenter randomized trial in orthopedic surgery. *Control Clin Trials;* 24(6):719–725.

8. Hannan EL, Racz M, Kavey RE, et al (1998) Pediatric cardiac surgery: the effect of hospital and surgeon volume on in-hospital mortality. *Pediatrics;* 101(6):963–969.

9. Kreder HJ, Deyo RA, Koepsell T, et al (1997) Relationship between the volume of total hip replacements performed by providers and the rates of postoperative complications in the state of Washington. *J Bone Joint Surg Am;* 79(4):485–494.

10. Schmidt CM, Turrini O, Parikh P, et al (2010) Effect of hospital volume, surgeon experience, and surgeon volume on patient outcomes after pancreaticoduodenectomy: a single-institution experience. *Arch Surg;* 145(7):634–640.

11. Showstack JA, Rosenfeld KE, Garnick DW, et al (1987) Association of volume with outcome of coronary artery bypass graft surgery. *Scheduled vs nonscheduled operations. JAMA;* 257(6):785–789.

12. Sosa JA, Bowman HM, Gordon TA, et al (1998) Importance of hospital volume in the overall management of pancreatic cancer. *Ann Surg;* 228(3):429–438.

13. Sosa JA, Bowman HM, Tielsch JM, et al (1998) The importance of surgeon experience for clinical and economic outcomes from thyroidectomy. *Ann Surg;* 228(3):320–330.

14. Taylor HD, Dennis DA, Crane HS (1997) Relationship between mortality rates and hospital patient volume for Medicare patients undergoing major orthopedic surgery of the hip, knee, spine, and femur. *J Arthroplasty;* 12(3):235–242.

15. Bombardier C, Hayden J, Beaton DE (2001) Minimal clinically important difference. *Low back pain: outcome measures. J Rheumatol;* 28(2):431–438.

16. Roland M, Fairbank J (2000) The Roland-Morris Disability Questionnaire and the Oswestry Disability Questionnaire. *Spine;* 25(24):3115–3124.

17. Okike K, Kocher MS, Mehlman CT, et al (2007) Conflict of interest in orthopedic research. *An association between findings and funding in scientific presentations. J Bone Joint Surg Am;* 89(3):608–613.

18. Bekelman JE, Li Y, Gross CP (2003) Scope and impact of financial conflicts of interest in biomedical research: a systematic review. *JAMA;* 289(4):454–465.

19. Cho MK, Shohara R, Schissel A, et al (2000) Policies on faculty conflicts of interest at US universities. *JAMA;* 284(17):2203–2208.

20. Krimsky S, Rothenberg LS (2001) Conflict of interest policies in science and medical journals: editorial practices and author disclosures. *Sci Eng Ethics;* 7(2):205–218.

21. Lo B, Wolf LE, Berkeley A (2000) Conflict-of-interest policies for investigators in clinical trials. *N Engl J Med;* 343(22):1616–1620.

22. McCrary SV, Anderson CB, Jakovljevic J, et al (2000) A national survey of policies on disclosure of conflicts of interest in biomedical research. *N Engl J Med;* 343(22):1621–1626.

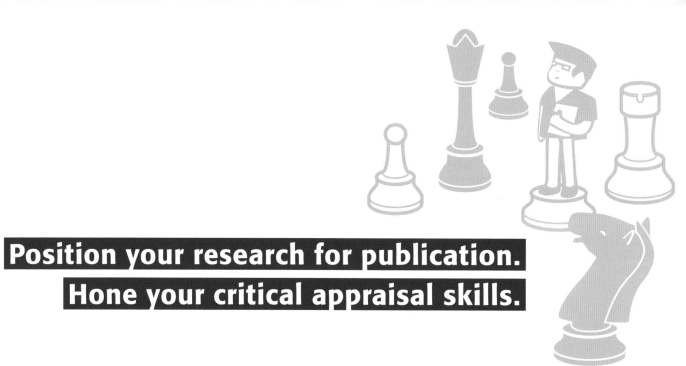

Position your research for publication.
Hone your critical appraisal skills.

9   Special topics

This chapter begins with practical advice on publishing your research. You will note that following the SMART-B approach positions your research nicely for the publication process. As with all SMART-B chapters, this section also assists you with honing your critical appraisal skills. Even if you never publish your study, you will need to be able to critically evaluate the literature in order to make the best treatment decisions for your patients. Special topics related to exploring which pa-tients may benefit the most or the least from procedures, in-formation on registries and their use, and the use of evidence in policy formulation provide you with insight on additional applications of the SMART-B approach for the creation and use of evidence. These sections provide food for thought for all researchers on some of the next phases for applying these concepts and the ramifications of producing or not producing high-quality studies.

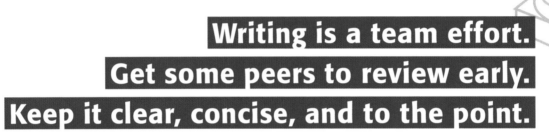

Writing is a team effort.
Get some peers to review early.
Keep it clear, concise, and to the point.

9.1　　Manuscript preparation:
being SMART about getting published

After you have developed your study questions and study plan, executed your study successfully, and performed the data analysis, it is time to get busy writing! Many investigators reach this point in the process so exhausted that they put the data aside and forget about it for a while. It is not uncommon to leave such a tremendous effort behind by failing to actually write the study manuscript. Continued discipline and perseverance is paramount for your hard work to have an impact on clinical practice. Unfortunately, we cannot just push a button and all our results, tables, and figures appear in manuscript format. This comes back to ensuring from the beginning that you have assembled a strong team for your study (large or small). You have adequately delegated and discussed the role of each investigator with respect to both authorship and writing responsibilities. By dividing up roles and sharing responsibilities for writing, the task becomes less daunting.

Most manuscripts can be divided into the following sections:

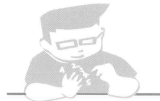

- Introduction
- Methods
- Results
- Discussion
- Conclusion

Keep in mind that each journal may have different requirements, and therefore the major sections may change slightly. However, these basic elements should be included in any study manuscript for publication. As a rule, it is often helpful to begin by writing the methods and results sections first, followed by the introduction and discussion sections. Generally, the abstract is written last, since this is meant to be a summary of the key points in your study. This chapter briefly summarizes the essential components of each of these sections and provides some insight about the manuscript submission process.

In addition to the material presented in this chapter, it is important to become familiar with the Consolidated Standards of Reporting Trials (CONSORT) 2010 Statement, which provides guidance for reporting on individually randomized, two group, parallel trials. In summary this chapter will cover many of these principles for all studies which include a diligent attention to clarity, completeness, and transparency of reporting. Being clear and not ambiguous will serve the interests of all readers. The CONSORT 2010 statement solely addresses the reporting of what was done and what was found (not design and execution). More information and a complete checklist is available through the CONSORT website (www.consort-statement.org).

9.1.1 Introduction

If your study was part of a grant application or had a formal study protocol associated with it, you can borrow from the background and significance sections of those documents when writing the introduction. However, make sure you have done an up-to-date literature search to identify any additional relevant articles that have been published since you started your study. It is important to keep your introduction relatively brief. The key is to inform the reader as to why your topic is important. It is not necessary to spend a tremendous amount of effort reiterating what others have already discussed in previous studies on your topic. Try to make your introduction interesting and to the point. The introduction should end with a clear and concise description of your study questions and objectives. If you have more than one question or a secondary question, list them separately. For an introduction to the case example on posterolateral fusion (PLF) and interlaminar lumbar instrumented fusion (ILIF) (chapter 2: Constructing a SMART study question), one possible structure could be:

1. Introductory paragraph on lumbar fusion with historical references to the performance and use of PLF.

2. Brief description of the ILIF procedure and its potential advantages and disadvantages compared with PLF.

3. A paragraph or statement on the dearth of quality literature examining ILIF. This is important because it is the reason why your comparative study is significant and worthy of readership. This also transitions nicely into the actual study objectives and methods.

In summary, consider these key elements in your introduction:

- Inform the reader as to why your topic is important.
- Report the potential clinical significance of your study, both in general terms and with particular reference to the specific goals and priorities of the intervention being studied.
- A statement regarding the novelty and impact of the work can also be helpful for the reader (and reviewer).
- Keep the literature review brief. Point out the gaps in the existing literature that your study may fill.
- Try to make the introduction interesting and to the point.
- End the introduction with a clear and concise description of your study questions and objectives.

9.1.2 Methods

This section is where you inform the reader about which study design you chose to answer your study questions. It also gives you the opportunity to describe the institutions in which you recruited your subjects. You get to tell the story of how you identified and recruited subjects, the characteristics of these subjects, how many participated, and how many you lost to follow-up. Describe the methods in sufficient detail so that the reader can reproduce your study. This section is typically divided into the following subsections:

- Study design
- Subjects
- Recruitment methods and data collection
- Measurements
- Data analysis plan

Study design
This subsection should be concise and to the point. Here specify whether your study was a randomized or quasi-randomized controlled trial, cohort study, case-control study, or case-series. Also mention here whether you used additional methods, such as matching, block randomization, stratified randomization, etc. More details on study designs can be found in chapter 4: Importance and implications of study design selection.

Subjects

Describing your study population clearly and thoroughly is important. Readers need to know if your results and conclusions can be generalized to other populations. Additionally, it is important to place your study in time. Technological advances, changes in patient care procedures, and differences in reporting practices at different times can affect the outcomes and interpretation of your study [1]. The following items should be included in this section:

- Explanation of inclusion and exclusion criteria
- Institutions in which you identified and recruited your subjects
- Time period in which you collected your data

For retrospective studies, give the dates during which the data were originally collected as opposed to when you abstracted them from the study.

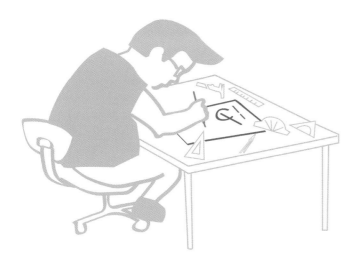

Recruitment methods and data collection

It is important in this subsection to describe clearly and concisely the process by which you identified and recruited subjects, and whether the subjects finished the study. Full accountability of every subject should be attempted. The follow-up procedures used in your study should be precisely defined as well. Did this involve an actual clinical assessment, a telephone interview, or an assessment of the clinical records? When possible, provide a schematic summary of the study showing the number and disposition of participants at each stage (**Fig 9.1-1**). The schematic summary should include:

- Total number of subjects approached
- Total number of subjects found eligible and ineligible
- Number of subjects who agreed to participate and signed an informed consent document
- Number of subjects who did not complete the study or did not have complete data (eg, lost to follow-up, withdrew, or died)
- Number of subjects who completed the study and whose data are included in the final analysis

Make every attempt to describe the following subjects:

- Screened, but did not meet the study criteria
- Approached, but declined to participate
- Enrolled, but were withdrawn or "dropped out"
- Enrolled, but were lost to follow-up
- Enrolled and completed the study

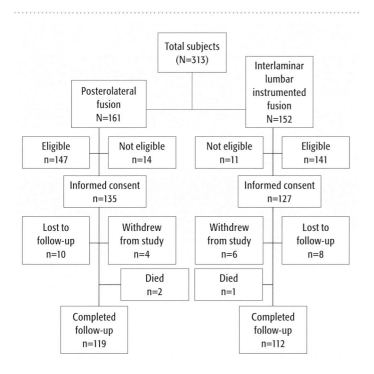

Fig 9.1-1 Example of a schematic summary of a cohort study (also known as a consort diagram).

Measurements

Baseline prognostic factors as well as intraoperative and outcome measurements that were collected should be described in this subsection of your study manuscript. If special measurements were used to define these, then you must identify them, provide any background information as to their validity, reliability, and responsiveness, and if appropriate, provide a copy of the measurement in your manuscript. A clear description of the measurement's content, scale, and interpretation with appropriate references should be included, regardless of whether you provide an actual copy of the measurement. More details on measurements are provided in chapter 5: Measurements.

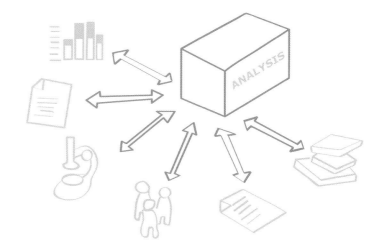

Data analysis plan

The overall intent of statistical reporting can be summarized this way: "Describe statistical methods with enough detail to enable a knowledgeable reader with access to the original data to verify the reported results" [2]. This subsection should provide a clear and concise description of how you analyzed your data so that others can repeat it.

☞ **The most readable and understandable data analysis subsections are those that reiterate their objectives and ensure that the data analysis plan maps directly onto your study objectives.**

The reader should be able to read the objectives and understand clearly what analysis was used to meet those objectives. It is not uncommon to get lost in the murkiness of an analysis section and forget the overall purpose of the study or intended objectives. By reiterating the objectives, readers can confirm that the overall plan and purpose of the study were executed. It is also a good idea in this subsection to reiterate your power calculations to validate whether you achieved the necessary number of patients in your study. Finally, identify the statistical package or program (with its corresponding reference) used to analyze the data. Results may vary slightly from package to package due to discrepancies in validation and updating.

9.1.3 Results

For the sake of brevity, the results section should not offer too much explanation or justification for your study's findings. This should be done in your discussion section. The flow of the results section should begin with descriptive statistics of the study groups, findings with respect to baseline, and intraoperative measurements with an accompanying table, which is typically the first table in your manuscript. Using the PLF and ILIF case example, **Table 9.1-1** provides an example of such a table.

	PLF		ILIF	
	No. or mean	% or range	No. or mean	% or range
Age (years)	63 (mean)	52–72	65 (mean)	50–69
Gender (female)	55	46%	50	45%
L4/5	80	67%	70	63%
L3/4	30	25%	30	27%
L2/3	9	8%	12	11%
Spondylolisthesis, grade I	90	76%	100	89%
Spondylolisthesis, grade II or above	29	24%	12	11%
Diabetic	25	21%	27	24%

Table 9.1-1 Baseline data for chronic low back pain patients treated with PLF and ILIF.

From this table, we note that both groups are relatively equal with respect to age, gender, diabetes, and surgical level. However, if we examine the distribution of spondylolisthesis severity, we observe that the ILIF group had a higher proportion of grade I spondylolisthesis treated than the PLF group. If the treatment of grade I spondylolisthesis is associated with a better outcome than higher-grade spondylolisthesis in general, then this disparity between groups may confound the conclusions that can be drawn. An unequal distribution between treatment groups of an independent factor that is also associated (negatively or positively) with the outcome constitutes a potential confounding variable. Potentially confounding variables should be dealt with in the analysis. Eliminating bias is covered in chapter 8: Bias reduction.

The descriptive section is then followed by the analytical sections where you should reiterate your objectives by using subheadings with sections that answer each objective separately. This allows the reader to follow the flow of your study manuscript from the objectives to the analysis plan, and then onto the results, without getting "lost in the weeds" so to speak. The effective use of tables and figures is key to presenting the results effectively. Complex numerical data are usually best presented in a table, while graphs are effective in illustrating differences between groups. Avoid presenting similar data in both tables and figures. The selective use of clinical photographs, intraoperative visuals, or imaging studies can effectively illustrate key points and can make the article interesting and readable. A more detailed discussion on descriptive and analytical statistics can be found in chapter 6: Analysis.

9.1.4 Discussion

Since the results section is intended to report your findings without interpretation, the discussion section allows you to put your findings in context.

The discussion section has a tendency to take on a life of its own. It is common for this section to become long and difficult to read.

It is also common for this section to serve as a platform for the author to give their opinions with respect to the treatment intervention being evaluated. Some go as far as to discuss public policy changes in their discussion. There are no specific, standard guidelines for this section, which is probably why authors take the liberty to write everything they were not able to write in the previous sections of the manuscript. Be careful with this approach. It is refreshing to read a discussion that is clear and concise. If you present your methods and results in an effective way, then the discussion allows you to interpret those results in such a way as to allow the readers to make up their minds in the end.

In order to help you avoid the temptation of writing too much with too little substance, here are some suggested steps for writing the discussion section:

1. Discuss the implications of the primary analyses first.
   – Secondary analyses should be discussed later and described as explanatory.
   – The opening paragraph should summarize the key findings and clinical significance of these results.

2. Distinguish between statistical and clinical significance.
   – Statistical significance relates to how likely the observed effect is due to chance (ie, sampling variation).
   – Clinical significance relates to the magnitude of the observed effect.

3. Discuss any weaknesses and strengths in your study design or problems with data collection, analysis, or interpretation.
    –   Disclosure of weaknesses or limitations is often difficult. However, honesty is the cornerstone of clinical research.
    –   Readers will often identify these weaknesses anyway, so discussing them gives you an opportunity to address them and recommend ways to overcome them when others attempt to answer similar questions.

4. Discuss your results in the context of the published literature.
    –   Describe the similarities and differences of your work with that of other authors who have done similar studies. Make an attempt to explain why your findings may be similar and/or different.
    –   Do not attempt to review the whole body of literature on this topic. Again, brevity is important, so be selective in which studies you choose to review.

5. Discuss the generalizability of your results.
    –   The purpose of your study is to produce results that the entire orthopedic, neurosurgical, and spinal communities can apply to their practice.
    –   The ability to generalize your findings is dependent on your study population, its inclusion and exclusion criteria, and other factors, such as your follow-up rate.

6. Remember that each paragraph of the discussion should present one key idea or concept.
    –   The use of subheadings can be an effective way to organize the flow of the discussion.

9.1.5 Conclusions

Limit your conclusions to only those supported by the results of your study. Unsupported conclusions are common in scientific research. Consider the following principles [1]:

*   You should provide equal emphasis on positive and negative findings.
*   Results of secondary or post hoc analyses should be presented as explanatory.
*   Conclusions should be based on fact and logic, not supposition or speculation.
*   Studies using surrogate end points (eg, muscle strength, range of motion, bone union) should be interpreted with caution. In other words, just because patients have solid fusion of the treated level does not necessarily mean they have a good final outcome if they cannot perform daily activities.

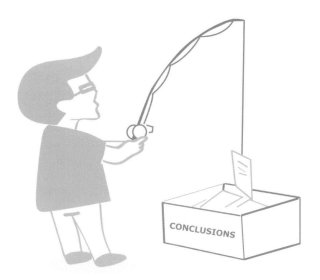

9.1.6 Submitting for publication

You have come to the end of a long journey. The study has been conceived, planned, executed, and analyzed. Your manuscript has been written. Now it is time to select a journal and submit your manuscript for publication. It is only through publication that you are able to help change or improve the way spine surgery is performed today. Regardless of whether your results are what you expected or wanted, publishing is important. Avoid the temptation to not submit results that are negative or counter to your hypothesis, which is known as publication bias.

Before submitting for publication, it is important to have your peers review your manuscript. In fact, it is advisable to have multiple colleagues review your manuscript as you develop it. For example, you may want to have your methods section reviewed before you draft the results section, since changes in your methods section will undoubtedly affect the way you report the results. Expect this process to be lengthy. Time spent having your colleagues review your paper is time saved later on when you submit it to a journal. It may even be the difference between acceptance and rejection.

An important point to emphasize along these lines is reciprocity. If you are asking colleagues to review your manuscripts (whether they are coauthors or not), be willing to return the favor.

The following are some important principles that you should consider when submitting your manuscript for publication:

- Select a journal that is most appropriate in regard to the audience you want to reach.
  - This may be intuitive if you are comfortable with the literature.
  - You may want to look at the tables of contents from past journals and visit the websites of specific journals to determine their missions and interests.

- Consider writing to the editor of one or more journals to determine whether they are interested in publishing on your topic.
  - This is not required and you may not receive an answer. However, it does not hurt to try and may save you some time in the long run.

- Ensure that you strictly adhere to the formatting and submission guidelines of the selected journal.
  - Every journal is different. Sometimes the differences are obvious and other times subtle.
  - Print the guidelines from the website and use them as a checklist. Go over them several times.

- If rejected, do not be discouraged.
  - Your study question may not meet the interests or needs of that particular journal. In these cases, it does not matter how good your manuscript is.
  - If you are not given the opportunity to resubmit, accept this decision and move on to another journal.

- Expect criticism and improve your paper accordingly.
  - No manuscript is returned without criticism and editing.
  - It is not uncommon to receive lots of criticism and even be asked to re-analyze your data in a different way.
  - Be objective, talk to colleagues, and decide if the criticisms are warranted. Most of the time they are. Try and accommodate the reviewer; however, do not compromise the intent of your study.

- Do not be afraid to argue your case.
  - It is not uncommon for a reviewer to misinterpret or misunderstand your findings.
  - If you feel this has happened, just respond with a clear and concise explanation. You may need to augment your argument with more data or make slight adjustments to your manuscript for clarification.

- Persevere and be patient.
  - After acceptance, it may take several months before your manuscript is actually in print.
  - Consider this part of the process and continue on with more research!

Element	Description
Abstract	• All good abstracts have a structure. Include only the most important elements of the manuscript. It should match the concepts and results from the manuscript precisely. • "Structured abstracts" are those with a particular structure required by the journal editor. A structured abstract is divided into sections with headings in bold print. The journal will set the requirement on these headings and the word count.
Introduction	The key is to inform the reader as to why your topic is important. It is not necessary to spend a tremendous amount of effort reiterating what others have already discussed in previous studies on your topic. Try to make the introduction interesting and to the point.
Methods	
• Study design	Randomized controlled trial, prospective cohort study, retrospective cohort study, etc
• Subjects	– Explanation of inclusion and exclusion criteria – Institutions in which you identified and recruited your patients – Time period in which you collected your data
• Data collection	– A summary schematic and description outlining patients recruited, enrolled, lost to follow-up, and completed – Baseline and prognostic factors collected – Outcome measurements collected
• Data analysis	– Data analysis plan – Power analysis
Results	• Descriptive statistics • Analytical statistics
Discussion	• Discuss implications of primary analyses • Distinguish between statistical and clinical significance • Discuss study weaknesses and strengths • Discuss results within the context of existing literature • Discuss generalizability of results
Conclusions	Limit yourself to only those conclusions that are supported by the results of your study

Table 9.1-2 Example outline of a typical manuscript.

9.1.7 Summary

- Highlighting many of the important points summarized in this chapter, **Table 9.1-2** can be used as a checklist when preparing your manuscript.

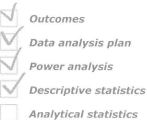
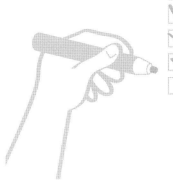

CHECKLIST

✓ *Outcomes*

✓ *Data analysis plan*

✓ *Power analysis*

✓ *Descriptive statistics*

☐ *Analytical statistics*

9.1.8 References

1. **Lang TA, Secic M (eds)** (1997) How to Report Statistics in Medicine. Philadelphia: American College of Physicians.
2. **International Committee of Medical Journal Editors** (1991) Uniform requirements for manuscripts submitted to biomedical journals. *N Engl J Med;* 324(6):424–428.

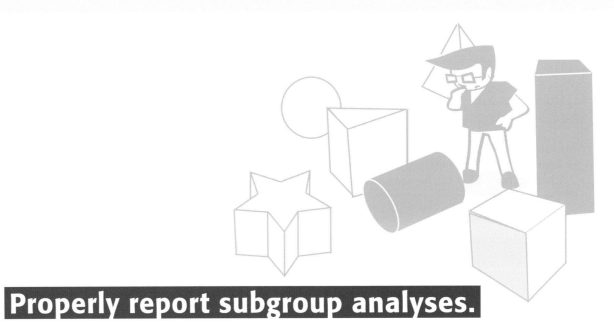

Properly report subgroup analyses.
Identify what is modifying the treatment effects.

9.2   Heterogeneity of treatment effects

9.2.1 Introduction

A clinical trial seeks to answer the question: "Is treatment A better than treatment B on average for a select population?" However, clinicians seek an answer to a different question: "Is treatment A better than treatment B for this specific patient?" The best treatment for a population may not be the same as for the individual patient, since the same treatment often produces different results in different patients. Some receive substantial benefits, many receive little or no benefit at all, and a few are even harmed by the treatment [1]. The term that describes this situation is the heterogeneity of treatment effect (HTE).

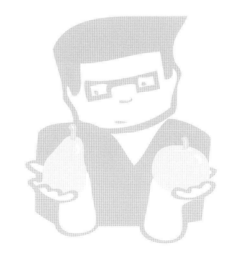

9.2.2 What factors influence heterogeneity of treatment effects?

There are several factors that can influence HTE. Kravitz et al [1] describe four of these factors:

- Risk of disease without treatment: This factor represents the prognosis of the patient who receives no treatment, a placebo treatment, or a standard (nonexperimental) treatment. It is similar to the natural history of the disease.
- Responsiveness to treatment: This factor relates to the probability that a patient will experience a benefit from the treatment. This can depend on many other factors, such as the technique of the surgeon, the effectiveness of an implant, or the concentration of a biologic at the target site.
- Vulnerability to adverse events: This factor is the likelihood that a patient will experience a side effect that would not occur in the absence of the treatment. Whether a patient experiences treatment-related or disease-related events will often depend on the context. For example, adjacent segment disease following fusion may be related to either the treatment or the disease.
- Utility for different outcomes: This factor reflects the importance that an individual patient places on the outcome. This often represents a compromise among different dimensions of quality and is patient specific.

9.2.3 How can heterogeneity of treatment effects be identified?

Heterogeneity of treatment effects can be identified by examining subgroups within a randomized controlled trial (RCT).

As an example, suppose there is an RCT comparing fusion with conservative care in patients with low back pain that is believed to be caused by degenerative disc disease. The outcome of the study is the proportion of patients who achieve a 50% improvement in pain over baseline after 1 year. In our hypothetical example, 26% in the fusion group achieved the desired outcome compared with 18% in the conservative group, with a risk difference of 8%, (95% confidence interval [CI]: -9–25%, $P = .23$) (**Fig 9.2-1**).

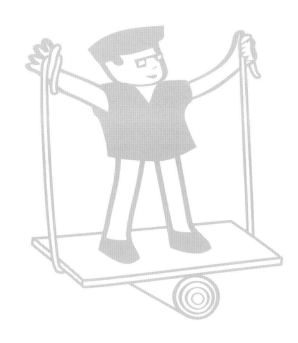

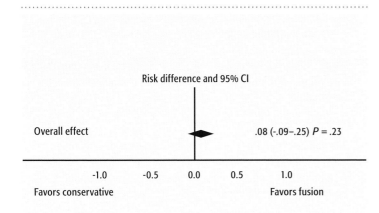

Fig 9.2-1   In this example, the solid vertical line represents the "null"—no difference between groups in the proportion of patients obtaining the desired benefit. The effect of treatment for all patients is represented by the diamond, the center representing the point estimate, and its horizontal tips representing confidence interval (CI). Statistical significance is achieved if the diamond lies completely to the left or right of the solid vertical line. In this example, there is no statistical significance between conservative care and fusion.

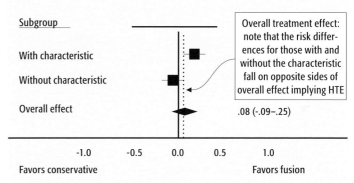

Fig 9.2-2   Stratifying the results on the presence and absence of an important characteristic produces a different picture than simply looking at the overall results. The dotted line represents the point estimate of the overall effect. Estimates in patients with and without the characteristic of interest are on opposite sides of the dotted line suggesting HTE, which should be confirmed by a statistical test of heterogeneity.

Now let us suppose there is a certain characteristic that a subgroup of patients possesses, which the investigators suspect influences the results. When the results are displayed based on the presence or absence of the characteristic, we see that those with the characteristic do better with fusion than with conservative care, while those without the characteristic do not (**Fig 9.2-2**). The differences between subgroups can be assessed statistically using a test of interaction. The interaction occurs between the treatment groups and the groups with and without the characteristic. When this happens, we say that the characteristic modifies the effect of the treatment.

9.2.4 Are there problems with identifying subgroups in randomized controlled trials?

👉 **Subgroup analyses are prone to spurious results due to the problem of multiple testing [2].**

Many caution against subgroup analyses, especially post hoc comparisons [3]. Nevertheless, identification of subgroup effects in clinical trials can generate important hypotheses about potential factors that modify treatment effects. When assessing subgroups, one should look for the following [3–5]:

- Statistical tests of interaction
- Description of whether the subgroup analysis was pre-specified or post hoc
- An incorrect inference that a subgroup effect (interaction) is present based on separate tests of treatment effects within each level of the characteristic of interest, ie, to compare one significant and one nonsignificant P value [6]

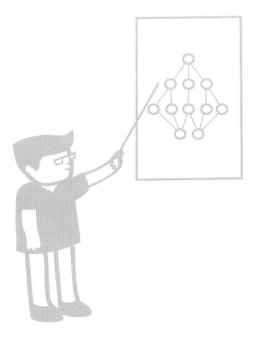

9.2.5 Summary

- Identifying characteristics that modify treatment effects is critical to patient-centered, individualized care.

- Proper reporting of subgroup analysis facilitates the recognition of patients who may respond better or worse than the average.

- Investigators conducting RCTs should consider characteristics that plausibly modify the effect of spine treatment. They should measure the appropriate characteristics, conduct subgroup analyses on those characteristics, and state their intentions to conduct subgroup analyses in their study protocol [3]. They should also consider increasing the sample size to assist in raising the power of the subgroup analyses.

- While it is important to not over interpret the results of subgroup analyses, it is necessary to recognize that HTE analyses assist in hypothesis generation and aids in the design of future confirmatory studies.

9.2.6 References

1. **Kravitz RL, Duan N, Braslow J** (2004) Evidence-based medicine, heterogeneity of treatment effects, and the trouble with averages. *Milbank Q;* 82(4):661–687.
2. **Brookes ST, Whitley E, Peters TJ, et al** (2001) Subgroup analyses in randomised controlled trials: quantifying the risks of false-positives and false-negatives. *Health Technol Assess;* 5(33):1–56.
3. **Moher D, Hopewell S, Schulz KF, et al** (2010) CONSORT 2010 Explanation and Elaboration: Updated guidelines for reporting parallel group randomised trials. *J Clin Epidemiol;* 63(8):e1–37.
4. **Gabler NB, Duan N, Liao D, et al** (2009) Dealing with heterogeneity of treatment effects: is the literature up to the challenge? *Trials;* 10:43.
5. **Wang R, Lagakos SW, Ware JH, et al** (2007) Statistics in medicine--reporting of subgroup analyses in clinical trials. *N Engl J Med;* 357(21):2189–2194.
6. **Matthews JN, Altman DG** (1996) Statistics notes. Interaction 2: Compare effect sizes not *P* values. *BMJ;* 313(7060):808.

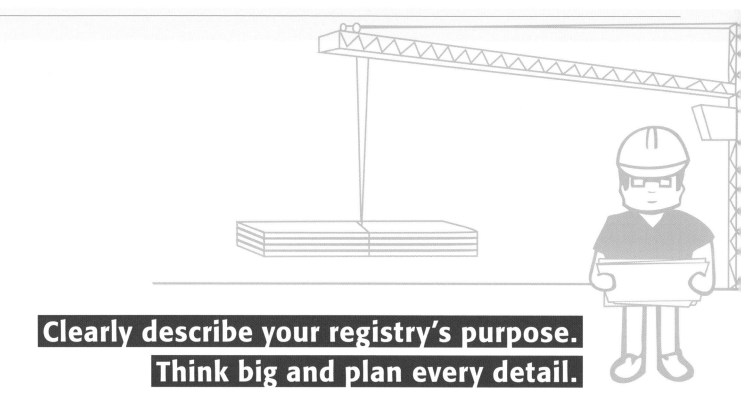

Clearly describe your registry's purpose. Think big and plan every detail.

9.3 Planning a SMART Registry

9.3.1 Introduction

The primary focus of this book is to assist spine surgeons in planning experimental and observational clinical studies. Within the continuum of clinical research is the prospect of creating a patient registry for observational or outcomes analysis. Prospective clinical studies, in particular randomized controlled trials (RCTs), are experiments typically designed to evaluate an intervention with strict inclusion and exclusion criteria, evaluating a homogeneous subject population. In contrast, registries are not typically designed to evaluate individual treatment comparisons (although specific treatments may be included in the registry) but rather observe the outcomes or natural history of several treatment options (including devices, drugs, and biologics), risk factors, and management strategies. Inclusion and exclusion criteria are typically much broader, which leads to a greater generalization of findings. Well-designed clinical studies are typically less prone to missing data and bias, and contain the risk factors and outcomes that are important to the researchers designing the study. On the other hand, registries are often challenged by missing data, poor follow-up rates, and sometimes, limited data on important risk factors or outcomes. No two registries are the same, nor should they be evaluated the same. Some registries violate many important evidence criteria vital in providing a respectable level of validity for making clinical decisions. However, many other registries are designed with the same rigor as a well-planned clinical trial.

This chapter provides an overview of the important criteria and phases of registry development. Following these criteria ensures that you design a high-quality registry. These same criteria can also be used to evaluate the quality of a registry or determine whether a specific registry has an adequate level of validity for answering an important clinical research question. Many concepts in this chapter are referenced from a guide published by the Agency for Healthcare Research and Quality (AHRQ) [1]. This publication provides key information on developing, operating, and evaluating registries. For individuals or groups interested in designing a registry, we highly recommend the second edition of this guide, which can be downloaded for free from the AHRQ website.

9.3.2 Purposes of registries

There are many purposes of a registry. The most common include:

- Describing the natural history of disease
- Determining the clinical effectiveness or cost-effectiveness of a drug, device, or process
- Measuring or monitoring the safety and harm of a drug, device, or treatment
- Measuring the quality of care

It is important that you clearly describe the purpose of your registry. Registries without a clear purpose are often not designed with sufficient focus and detail to answer pertinent questions. The purpose drives the planning, design, operations, and data analysis of the registry.

Sometimes a registry is not the best way to accomplish your goals. A clinical trial or simple retrospective study may suffice. For example, if you are interested in the comparative effectiveness of two treatments, or the effects of an important risk factor, designing a whole new registry for this alone is not worth the effort. Moreover, you may be able to answer your question with an existing registry. On the other hand, if your aim is to evaluate the long-term outcomes of a specific disease and include the risk factors, treatments, and outcomes where you may have multiple clinical questions, the design of a registry may be the best strategy. This should be considered first before embarking on such a large endeavor.

9.3.3 Planning a registry

Similar to a successful clinical trial, which is based on a well-written study protocol, every registry should have a guidance document or operations manual that outlines each critical area of registry planning and operations. This should be a living document that is continuously being developed as the planning progresses.

Some work can be done up front like the purpose and key questions, while other areas may evolve as you assemble a team of stakeholders to provide input on the development and future operations of the registry. The identification and commitment of stakeholders from multiple viewpoints (eg, physicians, epidemiologists, statisticians, hospital administrators, advocacy groups, and industry representatives) are critical in ensuring that you have a well-planned and thought-out registry, which will not need a major overhaul in the future.

When planning a registry, you can think of its development in four phases:

- Phase I: registry design and data element selection
- Phase II: pilot testing, data validation, and development of the final data collection tool
- Phase III: development of technical specifications, operations planning, and training
- Phase IV: registry rollout, oversight, and governance

There is certainly overlap among the phases and some benchmarks may be accomplished in a different order depending on the specific registry. However, these phases provide a basic structure for registry development.

Phase I: registry design and data element selection

The goals of phase I are to define the purpose and key study questions for the registry, identify the sources of data that will be collected to answer these study questions, and prepare for future pilot testing of the data collection tool. This is by far the most time intensive phase in the development of your registry. You will undoubtedly note that topics discussed elsewhere in this book are also applicable to developing and utilizing your registry.

Designing a registry

Once your overarching plan for a registry is established, you should follow these planning steps:

1. Design the registry with the highest level of scientific rigor. This begins with formulating and establishing key study questions that are measurable and answerable. Based on these study questions, a study design can be selected. This may simply be a cohort study design, a case-series design, or even a case-control design if the registry is based on the occurrence of specific events.

2. Clearly define the patients for study (ie, target population) and decide whether a comparison group is needed. Similar to a sample size calculation of a clinical trial, some thought should be put into determining how many patients need to be studied and for how long in order to fulfill your registry's purpose and answer the key study questions. This may include considering and specifying the magnitude of an expected clinically meaningful effect.

3. Establish an operations plan for data collection, data querying, and data entry. Essentially, this addresses how you are going to ensure that your data is of the highest quality and integrity, and that you have minimized missing values. This is an extremely important aspect of designing and maintaining a quality registry. In an ideal situation, the system in place should rival that of a prospective clinical trial with a certain level of monitoring and auditing.

4. Formulate a plan for where the data will be housed and how it will be managed, secured, and backed-up.

5. Consider what the potential sources of bias may be and how they will be handled.

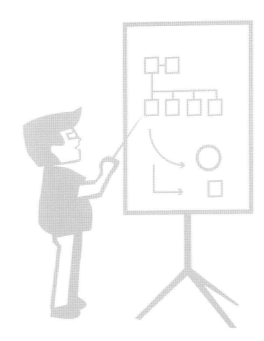

Data element selection

The data to be included in your registry depends in part on the source of your data. If you are designing a registry from scratch and your staff and staff from other sites are collecting the data prospectively, then you can choose which data elements you want to include. On the other hand, if you are getting your data from existing medical records or data warehouses, then you are constrained to what is available in those databases.

The initial selection of data elements should be based on your key study questions. If you are using existing data, you will need to determine if the available data elements will answer your key study questions. If not, you may have to modify those study questions.

The chosen data elements should be reliable (ie, repeatable) and valid (ie, represent what they are intended to represent). Related to validity is the issue of missing data, especially for follow-ups. High rates of missing data may invalidate the findings that you report. Sometimes you need to exclude an important data element when the percentage of missing data is too high. Consider missing data rates of greater than 20% as a significant threat to the validity of your results.

Another important question to consider is the time and cost involved in either obtaining the existing data or in collecting primary data. Determine the different sources of data and the feasibility of obtaining these data from existing databases, additional clinical templates, and so on. When collecting primary data, you need to consider the burden on the clinician or study coordinator as well as on the patients.

Once these large issues have been considered, then the stakeholders can move forward and list all potentially important data elements. These should be divided by exposure and outcome variables. They can be categorized by domains, such as sociodemographic, disease, general health, psychosocial, and outcomes variables.

Validated outcome measurements should be considered first if they are applicable to your patient population and study questions. A comprehensive literature search to identify valid, reliable, and responsive measurements should be considered. You can also reference books on spine disease severity measures, measurements, and outcomes to gain a comprehensive view of existing measurements and their overall content and quality [2, 3]. For example, the National Neurosurgery Quality and Outcomes Database registry for spine surgeries include in their outcomes questionnaire the Visual Analogue Scale (VAS), Oswestry Disability Index (ODI), Euro-Quol 5D (EQ-5D), and the North American Spine Society's Patient Satisfaction Index (PSI).

The clinical utility of measurements used in a registry should also be considered. Clinical utility can be evaluated based on patient and clinician friendliness [2, 3]. With respect to whether an instrument is deemed patient friendly, consider the following questions:

- Can the instrument be completed in a relatively short time?
- Are the questions clear, concise, and easy to understand?
- Will patients be uncomfortable answering the questions?

With respect to whether an instrument is deemed clinician friendly, consider the following questions:

- Is this instrument completed by the staff or self-administered?
- What is the staff effort and cost in administering, recording, and analyzing?
- How much time is required to train the staff in administering the instrument?

The final selection of measurements should be based on a review of each measurement's content, methodology, and clinical utility, as well as based on pilot testing (see phase II). The success of measuring outcomes in a registry is predicated upon the selection of appropriate measurements as well as compliance in completing these measurements. In the end, stakeholders need to select the least amount of measurements to cover the overarching purpose and key study questions in order to avoid undue burden on all those involved.

Ultimately, you should create a data collection tool (paper form) for the primary data you will be asking clinical staff to collect. This is then sent around for internal review among the stakeholders to estimate the burden on patients and clinicians. Prior to formal pilot testing, it is advisable to send this for an outside review (validity testing) in the form of a draft data collection tool.

Operations planning

With respect to the data collection process and to ensure high levels of quality assurance, you need to consider the following:

- Where will the data be stored? How will security be ensured?
- Develop standard operating procedures (SOPs) for collecting, cleaning, storing, monitoring, reviewing, and reporting data.
- How are personnel trained?
- How are data problems handled (eg, missing, out-of-range, or illogical data)?
- Define all requirements for quality assurance based on:
  - Identifying the most important or likely sources of error
  - Potential lapses in procedures that may impact the quality of the registry

With respect to adverse event reporting, you need to consider the following:

- Develop a plan for detecting, processing, and reporting adverse events.
- Consider sponsor-mandated reporting requirements if applicable.
- Discuss with government regulators if this is related to a regulated device, drug, or biologic.

Several other important operational considerations are ethical and legal issues, government regulations (such as the Health Insurance Portability Accountability Act [HIPAA] in the United States), transparency of activities, a registry oversight plan, and data ownership. Furthermore, like a clinical trial, you need to consider patient and provider recruitment and management. Factors that influence participation in a registry include:

- Perceived relevance
- Perceived importance
- Scientific credibility
- Risks and burdens of participation
- Incentives for participation

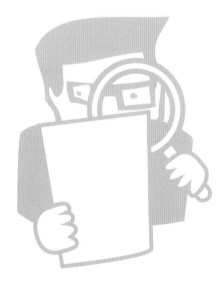

Analysis and interpretation of registry data

Similar to a study protocol, a clear and concise analysis plan should be created before the registry becomes operational. Areas to consider include:

- Completeness of data and data quality
- Procedures for handling and reporting missing data
- Patient population, the exposures of interest, and end points
- Is this registry descriptive or analytical, or both?
- Generalizability of the target population to the greater population

There should be a plan for how often data are reviewed for quality assurance and how often data are accessed for descriptive and analytical purposes. A well-thought-out registry will even consider describing the different tables and reports that will be produced on a regular basis.

At the completion of phase I, you should have a draft guidance document that details the areas discussed earlier and includes a draft protocol suitable for submission to an institutional review board (IRB) or ethics committee.

Phase II: pilot testing, data validation, and development of the final data collection tool

The goals of phase II are to conduct a pilot test of the data collection tool, gauge the burden on patients and clinicians, assess the validity of data obtained from existing databases, and finalize the data elements. This begins with developing a pilot test assessment tool that evaluates, at a minimum, the following criteria:

- Time to completion
- Completeness of data
- Usefulness of data
- Patient burden
- Clinician burden
- Oversight and governance burden

Once this tool is developed and approved by stakeholders, then you can conduct your formal pilot test at your site or at multiple centers if you are developing a multi-site registry. Going into the detailed operations of a pilot test is beyond the scope of this chapter, however, a careful plan should be executed.

After the pilot test is completed, you should conduct an after-action review involving the stakeholders in order to evaluate the results of the pilot test and reevaluate the data collection tool. During this phase you should identify data quality from existing databases (eg, reliability, missing data, logical values) if you are using outside data sources. This also includes identifying data formats for primary data and existing databases to aid in analyses and reports. You should consider different study designs that might better help in the routine reporting of registry data to answer key study questions. You should also finalize the analysis plan (descriptive and analytical) in order to ensure that you are using appropriate methods to address the final data elements and answer the key study questions.

Phase III: development of technical specifications, operations planning, and training

The goals of phase III are to create the electronic template systems (if you use electronic medical records for capturing registry data), develop the plan and mechanism for data extraction from existing databases, and develop the patient enrollment, follow-up, and operations plan. The following checklist is a basic set of items that should be considered. Since each registry is different, we will not go into detail. However, this checklist should assist you in the planning for this phase.

- ☑ Work with information technology and database management personnel to development an electronic template system if you are capturing data through electronic medical records
- ☑ Develop the plans and extraction technology for obtaining all data from existing databases
- ☑ Design a patient identification and enrollment plan including enrollment strategies, screening and enrollment logs, etc
- ☑ Develop a final visit report form to capture reasons why a patient has left the registry (eg, death, loss to follow-up, discharged)
- ☑ Finalize and submit for approval the scientific registry protocol that will drive the conduct of operations, oversight, human subject issues, analyses, and reporting
- ☑ Write a communication report for participating centers describing the registry's relevance, trust with data, risks, estimated effort, and potential disruption of staff roles
- ☑ Finalize SOPs and registry manual for describing data-quality assurance measures (eg, logic checking, missing values), oversight, and strategies for retention consistent with the registry protocol

Phase IV: registry rollout, oversight, and governance

The goals of phase IV are to plan for ongoing registry oversight and governance, train staff to comply with the registry data collection requirements, and finalize the plan for how an investigator will access and utilize data from the registry. Once these items are in place and full IRB approval is obtained, then you can formally launch your registry.

The importance of data collection in the field of spine cannot be understated. Over the past two decades, there has been a 300% increase in the number of low back surgeries performed and a corresponding increase in the incidence and prevalence of lumbar fusions [4–6]. The data typically reported vary widely in the literature, with benchmarks based on tightly controlled studies, such as RCTs that may not necessarily reflect the real world environment. Data collection from registries may result in a method to assess quality and comparative effectiveness of spinal treatments in a heterogeneous population and an appropriate risk adjustment.

If you do not wish to undertake the development of a local registry, consider enrolling in a national registry. There are national aggregates of outcomes data obtained via a continuous national clinical registry, such as those for neurosurgical procedures through the National Neurosurgery Quality and Outcomes Database developed by the American Association of Neurological Surgeons and thoracic surgical procedures through the Society of Thoracic Surgeons database.

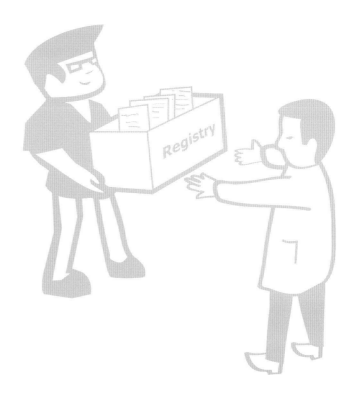

9.3.4 Summary

- Development of a registry is no small task. It requires a diverse group of collaborators, stakeholders, and often multiple sites to obtain acceptable patient numbers. Planning often exceeds that of a multi-site clinical trial.

- **Table 9.3-1** is a checklist that contains most of the criteria discussed in this chapter. This can be used as a resource for developing a patient registry.

- If you are considering using a registry to answer important clinical questions or evaluating a registry for critical appraisal purposes, we have also included a critical appraisal checklist for evaluating the overall validity by rating the registries level of evidence (**Table 9.3-2**).

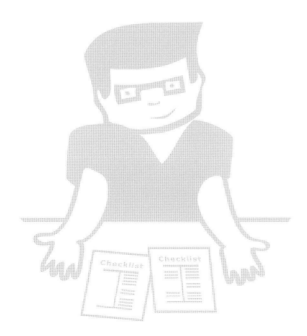

Registry development criteria	Completed	
	Yes	No
Planning		
Purpose		
Stakeholders and team		
Feasibility		
Funding		
Governance and oversight		
Goals for recruitment, retention, follow-up		
Design		
Study questions		
Study design		
Target patient population		
Data location		
Target number of subjects		
Potential sources of bias		
Data elements		
Relevant domains identified		
Baseline measurements		
Outcomes measurements		
Pilot test burden, accuracy, missing data		

Registry development criteria	Completed	
	Yes	No
Data sources		
Primary data collection		
Secondary data sources		
Ethics		
HIPAA, data ownership, etc		
Patient and provider recruitment and management		
Recruitment plan		
Strategy for enrollment and retention		
Data collection and quality assurance		
Data storage and data security		
SOPs for operations, data management, storage, and reporting		
Training of personnel		
Analysis and reporting		
Descriptive or analytical (or both) registry?		
Handling of missing data		
Frequency of reporting and by whom?		

Table 9.3-1 Checklist for registry development.

Studies from registries	
Study design	**Criteria**
Good quality registry	• Designed specifically for conditions evaluated
	• Primary data collected in a prospective fashion*
	• Process for monitoring quality of data
	• Patients followed long enough for outcomes to occur
	• Independent outcome assessment†
	• Complete follow-up of > 85% of patients
	• Controlling for possible confounding‡
	• Accounting for time at risk§
Moderate quality registry	• Prospective data from registry designed specifically for conditions evaluated
	• Absence of two other criteria for a good quality registry
Poor quality registry	• Prospective data from registry designed specifically for conditions evaluated
	• Absence of three or more other criteria for a good quality registry
	• Retrospective data or data from a registry not designed specifically for conditions evaluated

Table 9.3-2 Definitions of the different levels of evidence for registry studies.
* As opposed to accessing existing databases, medical records, or other secondary sources.
† Outcome assessment is independent of healthcare personnel judgment. Some examples include patient reported outcomes, death, and reoperation.
‡ Authors must provide a description of robust baseline characteristics, and control for those that are unequally distributed between treatment groups.
§ Equal follow-up times or for unequal follow-up times in a survival analysis, accounting for time at risk.

9.3.5 References

1. **Gliklich RE, Dryer NA** (2007) *Registries for Evaluating Patient Outcomes: A User's Guide.* 1st ed: Rockville: Agency for Healthcare Research and Quality.
2. **Chapman JR, Dettori JR, Norvell DC (eds)** (2009) *Spine Classifications and Severity Measures.* Stuttgart New York: Thieme Publishing.
3. **Chapman JR, Hanson, HB, Dettori JR, et al (eds)** (2007) *Spine Outcomes Measures and Instruments.* Stuttgart New York: Thieme publishing.
4. **Ragab A, Deshazo RD** (2008) Management of back pain in patients with previous back surgery. *Am J Med;* 121(4):272–278.
5. **Weiner DK, Kim YS, Bonino P, et al** (2006) Low back pain in older adults: are we utilizing healthcare resources wisely? *Pain med;* 7(2):143–150.
6. **North RB, Kidd D, Shipley J, et al** (2007) Spinal cord stimulation versus reoperation for failed back surgery syndrome: a cost effectiveness and cost utility analysis based on a randomized, controlled trial. *Neurosurgery;* 61(2):361–369.

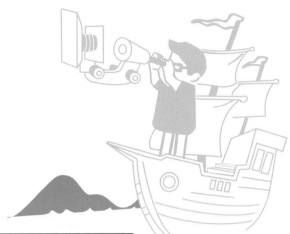

Pursue the highest quality of evidence.
Putting the clinical results in context.

9.4　Systematic reviews, comparative effectiveness, and health technology assessments

---

9.4.1 Introduction

Systematic reviews (SR), comparative effectiveness reviews, and health technology assessments (HTA) facilitate evidence-based practice and assist busy clinicians by providing a synthesis of research across a large number of studies on a given topic. They are used increasingly to form the basis for clinical practice guidelines, healthcare policy, and reimbursement.

This subchapter provides an overview of these types of evidence-based reports and additional resources for learning more about them. Evidence-based medicine (EBM) "requires new skills of the physician, including efficient literature searching and the application of formal rules of evidence in evaluating the clinical literature" [1]. This book provides you with many of these "new" skills.

9.4.2 Some history and perspective

In 1992, a "new paradigm for medical practice" was described in the Journal of the American Medical Association [2]. Moving away from "intuition, unsystematic clinical experience, and pathophysiologic rationale as sufficient grounds for clinical decision making", this new paradigm marked the emergence of EBM or evidence-based practice (EBP)—the systematic examination of findings from clinical research and their application to clinical practice. Evidence-based medicine is intended to complement clinical practice and enhance clinical decision making. Evidence-based practice then is the integration of the best research evidence with clinical expertise and patient values and preferences. Some of the earliest arguments in the 1990s for an evidence-based approach to medical practice were in the context of systematic development of clinical practice guidelines [1].

Archie Cochrane, a British physician for whom the Cochrane Collaboration is named, suggested in his 1972 book that since resources would always be limited, they should be used to equitably provide healthcare services shown to be effective in rigorously designed evaluations [3]. He emphasized the importance of using evidence from randomized controlled trials (RCTs) because these were likely to provide much more reliable and less biased information than other sources of evidence. His approach has been widely embraced by a number of professional and health policy circles as the gold standard of evidence available in clinical research (**Fig 9.4-1**).

Systematic reviews and meta-analyses have become mainstays in EBM. Particularly in the last decade, they have become the basis for the development of clinical guidelines, comparative effectiveness research (CER), and HTAs, in addition to facilitating evidence-based decision making with individual patients. The Institute of Medicine (IOM) has published standards for developing clinical guidelines, at the heart of which is performing an SR [4, 5]. The IOM has also published standards for conducting SRs [6]. The terminology related to SRs, CERs, and HTAs is somewhat confusing and there is significant overlap in concepts applied to all these [7].

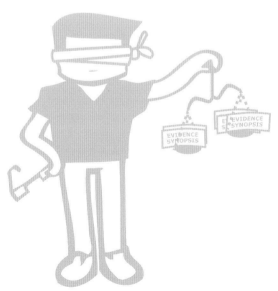

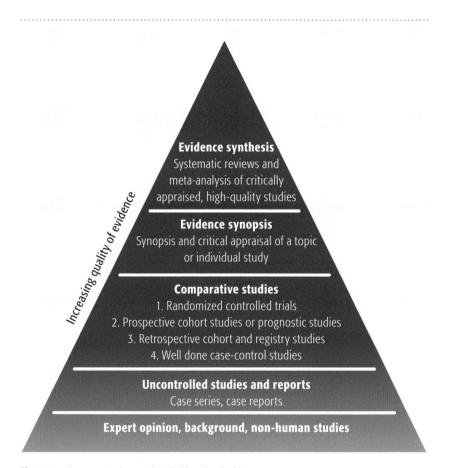

Fig 9.4-1   One conceptual approach to the hierarchy of evidence.

9.4.3 What is a systematic review?

Development of a formal SR has been an important part of advancing evidence-based decision making on numerous levels, including the formulation of clinical guidelines.

A systematic review is more than a summary or review of clinical literature. Ideally, an SR provides a comprehensive critical appraisal and synthesis of pertinent research studies on a specific clinical issue. Systematic reviews are the result of a planned, orderly, and methodical approach to searching for pertinent literature and synthesizing the highest-quality information from clinical studies to answer specific key questions.

Key questions in SRs can be related to treatment comparison, diagnosis or prognosis. Methodologically rigorous SRs form the basis for clinical practice guideline development, CER, and HTA.

On the surface, it may seem that performing an SR is simpler than designing and implementing clinical research. However, you should not underestimate the time, attention to detail, and focus needed to plan for and develop a high-quality SR. Depending on the scope and purpose of the SR, it may take many months to plan, execute, and report. The IOM has published a comprehensive set of standards for conducting and reporting SRs [6]. An indepth description of how to perform a high-quality SR is beyond the scope of this book; however, the IOM report is a comprehensive resource for the interested reader. Based on these resources, the general steps laid out in **Table 9.4-1** form the basis for performing an SR.

The majority of review articles searchable on PubMed are narrative reviews (NRs) rather than SRs, even though they may be listed as SRs. Generally, NRs are summaries of selected literature that describe and discuss the current state of the science on a particular topic or theme from a contextual or theoretical perspective. They may cover a wider range of issues for a given topic than an SR. There may be general questions that are broad and qualitative in nature that form the focus of the NR. Unlike SRs, they do not describe or follow a specified methodology for searching literature sources or inclusion and exclusion of literature that would permit replication to answer a specific quantitative research question. They may or may not provide formal critical appraisal of the validity of included literature. There is potential for bias in study selection and reporting, and inferences from NRs are generally not considered evidence based. The extent to which formal methods and procedures are described and followed in the review is a primary key to distinguishing SRs from NRs. Both have a role in the medical literature and it is important to distinguish between them.

1.	**Develop your rationale**	Before initiating an SR, there are some questions to consider up front about your topic: • Is there a need for a comprehensive review of the evidence? • What is the rationale for performing the review? Why is it needed? • What is the purpose of the SR? • What audience will it serve and how will it be used for decision making?
2.	**Formulate your topic**	Topic formulation should include a description of: • How an intervention (or risk factor) may be linked to the outcomes of interest. • If the topic relates to diagnostic testing, what is the clinical decision-making pathway? • What other tests are used in conjunction with or instead of it? • What is the next step for all possible outcomes (eg, true positive results) from doing the test? Such an analytic framework assists in defining the key study questions to be addressed. Each of the key study questions should be articulated in a standard format and the underlying rationale for each provided.
3.	**Design an appropriate protocol**	As with any research project, a protocol for conducting and reporting information in the SR is needed up front and should stipulate the following: • The context and rationale for the report as well as the timetable for completing it. • A population, intervention, comparison, and outcomes (PICO) table, or a population, prognostic factors, and outcomes (PPO) table that specifies the population, interventions, comparators, important outcomes, and relevant time points. Explicit inclusion and exclusion criteria for each component should be articulated a priori and included with your PICO/PPO table. The prespecified criteria should also describe study designs or features that should or should not be considered for inclusion. This serves as the basis for your literature search and establishes the criteria for screening and selecting studies for inclusion. • Search strategy, databases (including gray literature) to be searched, methods for identifying relevant evidence, and processes for documenting the search process. Separate search strategies may be needed for each key question. • Procedure for study selection including the screening process for participants, and the procedure for resolving disagreements between investigators. • Processes that are in place to diminish the introduction of bias into the selection, analysis, and reporting. • A data abstraction strategy and processes for managing data collection and analysis. • Critical appraisal methods to be applied to individual studies and how the overall body of evidence will be evaluated. • Describe and provide rationale for any planned analyses, including meta-analyses and explorations of differential effectiveness or safety in subgroups. • A report template or outline that describes how the various components and processes should be documented. • Identification, specification, and management of any conflicts of interest.
4.	**Perform a comprehensive literature search**	A structured, systematic search of the literature using the appropriate databases is then conducted based on the PICO/PPO table in order to identify potentially relevant publications for inclusion.
5.	**Select studies**	Selection of studies based on pre-established criteria and methods outlined in the protocol is carried out and documented.
6.	**Perform data analysis**	The data available is analyzed and synthesized within the context of study quality.
7.	**Assess the level of evidence**	Assessment of the overall strength of the body of evidence is made.
8.	**Report results**	A report is drafted that transparently documents the process followed and reports results in a clear and concise manner.

Table 9.4-1   General steps for performing a systematic review (SR) based on the Institute of Medicine (IOM) report.

9.4.4 What are comparative effectiveness research and health technology assessment?

Comparative effectiveness research and HTA are both geared toward informing healthcare policy.

☞ **Comparative effectiveness research compares interventions and strategies that prevent, diagnose, treat, or monitor health conditions. This type of research encompasses both the generation and synthesis of evidence. The intention is to assess a comprehensive array of information and data on health-related outcomes for diverse patient populations from a variety of data sources and study methods [8].**

The objective is to inform healthcare decisions by examining evidence on effectiveness, benefits, and harmful effects from different treatment options. Therefore, CER is generally broader than an SR, which may compare only two competing options. Two sources of evidence are extensive formal SRs, (comparative effectiveness reviews) of existing clinical studies, and studies designed to generate new evidence [9]. In general, before generating new evidence, a formal SR or comparative effectiveness review of what evidence currently exists can help identify gaps in knowledge and evidence, and help determine how to best address those gaps.The concept of CER is relatively new and continues to evolve. One notable development is the recent formation of the Patient-Centered Outcomes Research Institute (PCORI). The PCORI seeks to promote and fund CER, including evidence synthesis studies, with an explicit and core focus on questions that directly inform issues relevant to patients and caregivers. As such, all PCORI-funded projects require patient involvement at every stage of the project [10]. A partial list of selected resources for SRs, CER, and HTAs is available in **Table 9.4-2**.

Organization	Description of resources available
Agency for Healthcare Research and Quality (AHRQ) www.ahrq.gov	• Definitions and description of CER • Complete CER and HTA reports • Information on and link to clinical guidelines • Documents and training modules on methodology • Consumer materials and numerous other resources
Institute of Medicine (IOM) www.iom.edu	• Methodological guidelines for development of clinical guidelines and SRs
International Network of Agencies for Health Technology Assessment (INAHTA) www.inahta.net	• HTAs and economic analyses from over 50 agencies and 29 countries worldwide • Center for Reviews and Dissemination (CRD) database and NHS Economic Evaluation Database (EED) • Appraisal of economic studies is provided for EED citations • HTA glossary is a good resource for basic terminology
National Information Center on Health Services Research and Health Care Technology (NICHSR) www.nlm.nih.gov	• "HTA 101: Introduction to Health Technology Assessment" is a comprehensive monograph on the basic aspects of HTA, including aspects of economic analysis
The Cochrane Library www.theconchranelibrary.com	• Cochrane Database of Systematic Reviews • Cochrane Database of Methodology Reviews • Cochrane Central Register of Controlled Trials • Database of Abstracts of Reviews of Effects • Cochrane Methodology Register
Patient Centered Outcomes Research Institute (PCORI) www.pcori.org	• Background and research on the need for patient-centered outcomes • Funding opportunities

Table 9.4-2   Partial list of selected resources on systematic reviews (SRs), comparative effectiveness research (CER), and health technology assessments (HTAs).

The HTA process is usually initiated or commissioned by policy-making bodies with the explicit aim of informing policy decisions. Health technology assessments use SRs and comparative effectiveness review concepts and expand on them. As defined by the International Society for Pharmacoeconomics and Outcomes Research, HTA is "a form of policy research that examines short- and long-term consequences of the application of a health-care technology. Properties assessed include evidence of safety, efficacy, patient-reported outcomes, real-world effectiveness, cost and cost-effectiveness as well as social, legal, ethical and political impacts [11]." Not all components may be present in a single HTA report. Although thorough discussion of various components is beyond the scope of this book, it is worth highlighting some of them. These may also be part of SRs and comparative effectiveness reviews with the general exception of economic analyses.

Efficacy and effectiveness

Evidence of efficacy comes from RCTs. Although RCTs theoretically provide the least potential for biased results, they generally provide information about how the intervention works, usually in the short term (less than 24 months) and under ideal conditions in a selected group of patients (ie, "Can it work?"). Observational studies allow for evaluation of effectiveness (ie, "How does the intervention perform in more real-world circumstances?") and often provide more valuable information on long-term and rare outcomes (ie, "Does it work under usual clinical circumstances?").

Outcomes analysis

Systematic reviews, comparative effectiveness reviews, and HTAs all contain some analysis of how outcomes are the same or different between groups receiving alternative interventions. The analysis needs to go beyond reporting or considering statistical significance. The magnitude of the effects of a technology versus an alternative on the outcomes (benefits, harmful effects, and the benefit-risk ratio) must be considered. The directness of the outcome (ie, "Is it a patient-important outcome like death or a surrogate measure?") and the extent to which findings are clinically significant (ie, "Is there a minimal clinically important difference?") play important roles in evaluating the outcomes and assessing the body of evidence.

Cost and cost-effectiveness

In addition to establishing the efficacy and effectiveness of procedures, policymakers may also want to consider the economic impact of technologies. The most compelling economic analyses to payers are those that compare both the costs and efficacy of two competing options in a formal economic analysis. Such analyses require that efficacy has been established for both alternatives. Studies that report only costs, cost of illness, or do not compare alternatives are not considered full economic evaluations. Full economic evaluations identify and compare appropriate alternatives, their incremental impact on health outcomes, and their incremental costs. They conventionally compare two well-defined clinical alternatives in the form of an incremental cost effectiveness ratio (ICER), broadly defined as the cost per unit of clinical improvement. The ICER is derived by dividing the differences in effectiveness by the difference in costs. Terms related to economic evaluation are easily misused and misunderstood. **Table 9.4-3** provides a summary of the general types of economic studies.

Type of economic analysis	Effectiveness measurement	Outcome	Notes
Cost studies			
Cost only	None	Cost of procedure, treatment, or other charges	Can inform full economic evaluations
Cost of illness or economic burden	None	Includes indirect, patient, and/or societal costs	Can inform full economic evaluations
Full economic evaluations			
Cost minimization	Assumes equal effectiveness between alternatives	Difference in cost	Alternatives are rarely truly equal in effectiveness
Cost benefit	Costs of effects (benefits), costs of intervention	Net benefits, cost-benefit ratio, willingness to pay	Controversial to express benefits in monetary terms
Cost effectiveness	Natural or condition-appropriate measurement (eg, survival, pain reduction, time to recurrence)	Cost per improved outcome	Most useful for comparing studies that assess the same health state or condition, but less so for comparing studies of different health states
Cost utility	Quality-adjusted life-year (QALY) and disability-adjusted life-year (DALY)	Cost per QALY or DALY	Easiest to compare across studies and reflects more assumptions about the quality-of-life impacts of alternative therapies

Table 9.4-3   Summary of economic study types.

9.4.5 Statistical analyses

The nature of the literature and data available influences the type of statistical methods that are appropriate for SR, CER, and HTA. In some instances, only descriptive statistics are appropriate (chapter 6: Analysis), in other instances, simple pooling (weighted by sample size) may be appropriate. More advanced methods include meta-analysis and decision analysis, which may or may not be incorporated into SRs, comparative effectiveness reviews, and HTAs. Detailed descriptions of these methods are beyond the scope of this book.

Meta-analysis is the use of specific statistical methods for combining or pooling data from multiple studies in order to provide a quantitative estimate of the overall effect for a given outcome. Advantages to pooling data from studies using meta-analysis can include increasing statistical power for primary outcomes, assessing the variability across studies, enhancing the external validity of findings, identifying study characteristics that might influence the outcomes most, and potential resolution of uncertainty when reports disagree [12]. The factors that apply to creating a high-quality SR should be reflected in any meta-analysis. Statistical and methodological skill is required for performing a credible meta-analysis (chapter 9.5: Meta-analyses).

Pooling of data may not be appropriate and may provide misleading answers if clinical and statistical heterogeneity is not considered and explored. Including studies of different study designs (eg, case series combined with RCTs) or using sets of case series to compare treatments are generally not appropriate. In addition, the value of the pooled estimate of effect size for making conclusions can be severely limited by poor data quality in primary studies, bias in included studies, biased selection of studies, publication bias, or insufficient number of comparable studies. The quality of studies and data that you start with directly influences the quality and credibility of the meta-analysis.

Decision analysis is a method for breaking down a complex problem into components that can be analyzed in detail when there is uncertainty. It involves the modeling of alternative strategies (eg, decision to operate or not) in terms of the probabilities that specific events or outcomes will occur. Values or utilities (eg, average life years) are then specified for outcomes. Each decision is modeled (based on the probabilities and outcome values) and the results for each strategy compared [12]. Decision modeling can help clarify the dynamics and tradeoffs related to selecting one strategy over others. It is one type of quantitative modeling, and (as is the case with any modeling) assumptions and estimates used in the models need to be specified and transparent since they can greatly influence the results. While the results may be helpful in decision making, they should not be construed as statements of scientific or clinical fact [12]. Decision analysis may be used as part of economic modeling.

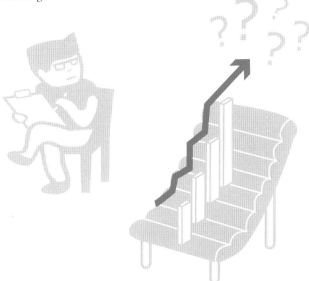

9.4.6 Critical appraisal of systematic reviews and meta-analysis

In many evidence pyramids describing the hierarchy of evidence, well-done syntheses of methodologically rigorous clinical studies are considered the highest level of evidence (**Fig 9.4-1**). However, not all SRs follow best practices for reducing bias or include the highest-quality studies.

☞ **A high-quality SR, comparative effectiveness review, or HTA follows specific methodologies, focuses on the highest-quality evidence, and critically appraises that evidence in order to put the results into context.**

Table 9.4-4 provides some general methodological principles to consider when reading any of these types of reports.

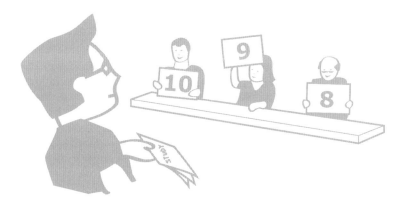

Methodological principle*
• Do the authors state the purpose, aim, study questions, and hypothesis?
• Was the literature search described and documented?
• Were inclusion and exclusion criteria stated a priori and followed?
• Are characteristics of included studies provided?
• Was the quality of included studies formally assessed and methods described?
• Was the overall quality of included studies given primary purpose?
• Was the overall strength of the evidence described?
• Were potential conflicts of interest stated?
Qualitative analysis
• Were studies appraised critically?
• Was the magnitude and direction of effect sizes evaluated?
• Was the consistency of effect sizes evaluated?
• Was the stability of effect sizes (eg, confidence intervals) evaluated?
• Was the scientific quality of studies considered in conclusions?
• Were methods to enhance objectivity incorporated?
Quantitative analysis (meta-analysis)
• Was heterogeneity evaluated?
• Was heterogeneity explored, if present?
• Were missing data handled appropriately?
• Were effect sizes pooled appropriately?
• Was a sensitivity analysis conducted?
• Was publication bias explored?
• Were potential sources of bias and limitations described?

Table 9.4-4   Methodological questions to consider when reading a systematic review. *Not all SRs include quantitative analysis, such as meta-analysis.

9.4.7 Impact on clinical practice and policy

Quality evidence syntheses, such as SRs (with or without me-ta-analysis), comparative effectiveness reviews, and HTAs are generally considered the highest quality of evidence in the evidence hierarchy (**Fig 9.4-1**). As previously mentioned, pay-ers and policymakers across the world have increasingly used evidence from these syntheses in their decision making. The quality of the evidence represented by the individual studies in such reviews directly impacts the overall quality and strength of the body of evidence. It is unfortunate that in many instanc-es the quality of evidence from clinical research published in the peer-review literature is poor. This makes decision making difficult and policy-making bodies may not approve the use of or reimbursement for a particular technology or procedure. This has been a source of frustration for clinicians who believe in the value of such technologies or procedures. It is up to the clinical research community to enhance the quality (and hence the credibility) of clinical research in order to support their beliefs and effectively make a case for their use with poli-cymakers. Although RCTs may not be possible or practical for a number of clinical and surgical situations, there are ways to improve the evidence via higher-quality research, regardless of study design. Applying the concepts in this book and seek-ing appropriate assistance with clinical study design, imple-mentation, analysis, and reporting are important steps.

9.4.8 Summary

Evidence-based practice is the integration of the best research evidence with clinical expertise and patient values and preferences. Systematic reviews, comparative effectiveness reviews, and HTAs facilitate evidence-based practice and assist busy clinicians by providing a synthesis of research across a large number of studies on a given topic.

- They are used increasingly to form the basis for clinical practice guidelines, healthcare policy, and reimbursement.

- They have many similarities but differ in scope and purpose. These are formal research studies that answer specific and focused key questions. All should follow a formal rigorous methodology for literature search and documentation, use pre-defined inclusion and exclusion criteria, perform formal critical appraisal of included studies, and synthesize evidence in a transparent, unbiased manner. Critical appraisal of these types of studies is important.

- The quality of the evidence represented by the individual studies in such reviews directly impacts the overall quality and strength of the body of evidence. Improving the evidence base via higher-quality research is needed, regardless of study design for many clinical topics.

- Quantitative synthesis of data, such as meta-analysis, may be part of a quality SR, comparative effectiveness review, or HTA.

- Full, formal economic analyses compare the incremental differences in both costs and efficacy for competing alternative treatments. Such studies are frequently part of HTAs and may be used for policy decisions. Studies that include costs only are not full economic studies.

9.4.9 References

1. **Eddy DM** (2005) Evidence-based medicine: a unified approach. *Health Aff (Millwood);* 24(1):9–17.
2. **Evidence-Based Medicine Working Group** (1992) Evidence-based medicine. *A new approach to teaching the practice of medicine. JAMA;* 268(17):2420–2425.
3. **Cochrane AL** (1972) *Effectiveness and Efficacy: Random Reflections on Health Services.* 2nd ed. London: Nuffield Provincial Hospitals Trust.
4. **Field M, Lohr KN** (1990) *Clinical Practice Guidelines: Directions for a New Program.* Washington, DC: National Academies Press.
5. **Graham R, Mancher M, Wohlman DM, et al** (2011) *Clinical Practice Guidelines We Can Trust: Standards for Developing Trustworthy Clinical Practice Guidelines (CPGs).* Washington, DC: National Academies Press.
6. **Eden J, Levit L, Berg A, et al** (2011) *Finding What Works in Health Care: Standards for Systematic Reviews. Washington, DC: National Academies Press.*
7. **Luce BR, Drummond M, Jönsson B, et al** (2010) EBM, HTA, and CER: clearing the confusion. *Milbank Q;* 88(2):256–276.
8. **US Department of Health and Human Services** (2012) Draft Definition of Comparative Effectiveness Research for the Federal Coordinating Council, Vol. *2012. Available at: www.hhs.gov. Accessed September 26, 2012.*
9. **Agency for Healthcare Research and Quality** (2012) What is Comparative Effectiveness Research? Vol. *2012. Available at: www.effectivehealthcare.ahrq.gov. Accessed September 26, 2012.*
10. **Selby JV, Beal AC, Frank L** (2012) The Patient-Centered Outcomes Research Institute (PCORI) national priorities for research and initial research agenda. *JAMA;* 307(15):1583–1584.
11. **Berger ML, Bingefors K, Hedblom EC, et al** (2003) *Health Care Cost, Quality, and Outcomes: ISPOR Book of Terms.* Lawrenceville: International Society for Pharmacoeconomics and Outcomes Research (ISPOR).
12. **Goodman CS** (2004) *HTA 101: Introduction to Health Technology Assessment.* U.S. National Library of Medicine. Falls Church: The Lewin Group.

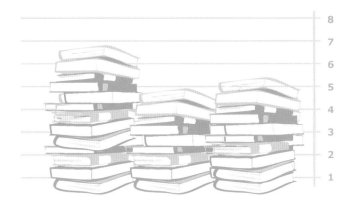

Meta-analysis is a powerful tool. Effect size does matter. Identify those confounders.

9.5   The SMART use of meta-analyses

9.5.1 Introduction

Meta-analysis is a statistical synthesis of related investigations that aims to determine if there is a significant effect and, if so, what the magnitude is of that effect. It assesses the variation within each study (heterogeneity) by measuring the consistency of results from study to study. The heterogeneity between studies may justify further investigation. Meta-analyses are best used to pool results of randomized controlled trials (RCTs). Other study designs can also be used, such as single-arm observational, prognostic, diagnostic test reliability, and cohort studies. This subchapter reviews the basic methodological techniques and how to interpret the results of meta-analyses.

Throughout this subchapter the following example, comparing vertebroplasty to nonoperative treatment, will be used to demonstrate how to perform and interpret a meta-analysis. A 75-year-old patient presents with a painful compression osteoporotic fracture, despite pharmacological management including opioids. She has significant functional lifestyle changes and poor sleep. She is asking whether a vertebroplasty will help and if it will last? In 2009, two articles published in the New England Journal of Medicine demonstrated no efficacy compared to sham, but other articles since those publications show an opposite outcome. How can this be interpreted to advise this patient?

9.5.2 Advantages of meta-analyses

👉 **Meta-analyses should be unbiased and based on the best available evidence. For this reason, meta-analyses are important in clinical and healthcare policy decision making.**

Other advantages include:
- Increasing statistical power: Combining similar studies into a meta-analysis can increase power and may show that a treatment is effective when several small studies fail to show statistical significance. In the example featured in **Fig 9.5-1**, two studies demonstrated a trend toward a greater relative risk of reoperation after fusion than arthroplasty at adjacent segments. This illustrates how pooling results with a meta-analysis reveals a significant effect is present.
- Improved generalizability: Meta-analyses examine generalizability since it includes studies from various investigators, usually with slightly different inclusion and exclusion criteria. This broadens the population for which results might apply.
- Focus on effect size: Individual studies are usually reported with tests of significance and *P* values, whereas meta-analyses evaluate effects sizes. The advantage of the latter being that this is a measure of the magnitude of effect.
- Subgroup analyses: Moderator variables and subgroup analysis in meta-analyses can be used to identify factors that explain variations between studies.

Study or subgroup	TDR Events	Total	Fusion Events	Total	Weight	Risk ratio M-H, Fixed, 95%CI	Risk ratio M-H, Fixed, 95%CI
Berg 2009	6	72	1	80	59.4%	6.67 [0.82–54.06]	
Guyer 2009	2	43	1	90	40.6%	4.19 [0.39–44.91]	
pooled	8	115	2	170	0.0%	5.91 [1.28–27.34]	
Total (95% CI)		115		170	100.0%	5.66 [1.16–27.58]	
Total events	8		2				

Heterogeneity: Chi² =0.09, df=1 (*P*=0.77); I²=0%
Test for overall effect: Z=2.15 (*P*=0.03)

0.01 0.1 1 10 100
TDR   Fusion

Fig 9.5-1   Pooled results of fusion versus total disc replacement (TDR) with the surgical treatment of adjacent segment pathology as the outcome. This example illustrates the effect of two randomized trials that are not statistically significant until they are combined. Combining studies increases statistical power and demonstrates a statistically significant difference. CI indicates confidence intervals.

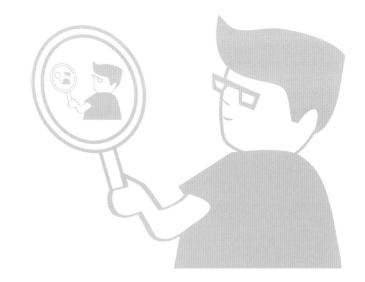

9.5.3 Limitiations of meta-analyses

- Meta-analysis can be performed even when only two studies are available, though they should be homogeneous. Most clinical studies, however, are heterogeneous. Therefore, small numbers of studies can lead to incorrect conclusions as the dispersion of error may be incorrectly predicted.
- Study designs, such as RCTs, are easily pooled in meta-analyses. Combining single-arm observational trials with RCTs may be problematic and should be done with caution. Problems may arise because the basic question is often different, and inclusion and exclusion criteria are expanded in observational studies.

A major weakness of meta-analysis is that it is only a statistical interpretation of studies and not a scientific investigation itself. It is subject to the many biases of the primary studies. Furthermore, weak studies result in poor meta-analyses. Most meta-analyses rely on published studies, which are biased for large effects size. Therefore, the meta-analysis may be biased in the same direction. Moreover, the individual performing the meta-analysis may have bias, which can affect which studies are included and the assumptions used in the meta-analysis. When reporting meta-analysis results, warnings regarding these limitations should be presented.

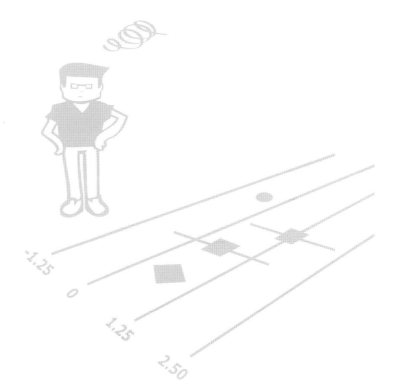

9.5.4 Validity of meta-analyses

Criteria for a valid meta-analysis are:
- Outcome of interest must be similar between studies (or at least measure the same domain) using comparable methods and procedures.
- Populations should be similar and free of bias selection.
- Predefined inclusion and exclusion criteria must be established, and all such studies are included. The systematic review should be transparent.
- Primary studies should be published in peer-reviewed journals, although it is acceptable to include regulatory reports, academic theses, or other unpublished studies. The effect of these nontraditional studies can be determined with a sensitivity analysis.
- Sensitivity analyses should be performed to examine how variation of key factors (such as inclusion criteria, choice of outcomes, and assumptions used in the meta-analysis) affect the statistical results.
- Studies should be evaluated for bias using objective instruments, such as the Review Manager software from the Cochrane Review.
- Publication bias assesses the possibility of missing or unpublished studies in the results. Studies with large effects can be eliminated to see if the results change in a significant way.

9.5.5 Meta-analysis methodology

The basic framework of a meta-analysis is a systematic review (**Table 9.5-1**). This topic is discussed in more detail in chapter 9.4: Systemic reviews. The systematic review starts with a study question, which is refined until it is succinct and clearly stated. This should be an important study question with clinical relevancy. A patients, intervention, comparison, and outcomes (PICO) table should be created so that the key study questions and variables to be studied are identified. Next a systematic literature search is performed and articles selected based on predefined inclusion and exclusion criteria. The data are abstracted and entered into a database.

In our vertebroplasty example, the key study question is: What is the safety and effectiveness of vertebroplasty compared to nonoperative treatment of painful osteoporotic compression fractures? A PICO table for this example has been constructed identifying the patient population, interventions, comparison, and outcomes (**Table 9.5-2**).

For our vertebroplasty example, a meta-analysis may have sufficient power to determine a true effect of vertebroplasty and help guide patient and surgeon decision making. After a systematic literature search, six RCTs were identified and data were extracted. Pain Visual Analogue Scale (VAS) and functional outcomes (Roland-Morris or Oswestry) were evaluated at early and late time points to evaluate adverse events and new secondary fractures.

SMART steps		Essential characteristics
S	Study question	• Should be developed and refined into a meaningful and succinct question
		• PICO table, outcome variables, time points
	Systematic review	• Transparent and unbiased
		• Establish inclusion and exclusion criteria
		• Search multiple databases
	Data abstraction	• Independently performed by two researchers
M	Meta-analysis	• Random versus fixed effects model
		• For each individual study, calculate standardized mean difference and confidence intervals
		• Pool data and calculate mean standardized difference and confidence intervals of all studies together
A	Analysis	• Test for significance
		• Assess heterogeneity (Q statistic, I^2)
		• Publication bias
		• Sensitivity analysis
		• Examine moderator variables and subgroups
R	Reporting	• Forest plots
		• Discuss causes of variance
		• Implications of effect size
		• Identify potential bias
T	Translate	• Interpret the findings in the context of the literature and translate to clinically relevant results

Table 9.5-1   Planning a SMART meta-analysis.

	Inclusion	Exclusion
Patient	• Symptomatic adult patients with osteoporotic compression fractures • Thoracic and lumbar spine • 1–3 levels • Low-energy fractures • No neurological deficits or complaints • Acute and subacute fractures less than 12 months old • Have not responded to at least 3 weeks of conservative treatment	• Patients younger than 60 years old • Cervical spine lesions • Patients with infection, tumor, and neuromuscular disease • History of cement augmentation
Intervention	• Vertebroplasty or kyphoplasty	
Comparison	• Sham injection • Standard nonoperative treatment	
Outcomes	• Pain Visual Analogue Scale (VAS) • Spine specific outcome (eg, Roland-Morris questionnaire, Oswestry Disability Index) • HRQOL (EQ5d, Qualeffo) • Adverse events • Secondary fractures	• Costs and cost-effectiveness measurements

Table 9.5-2   PICO table for vertebroplasty example.

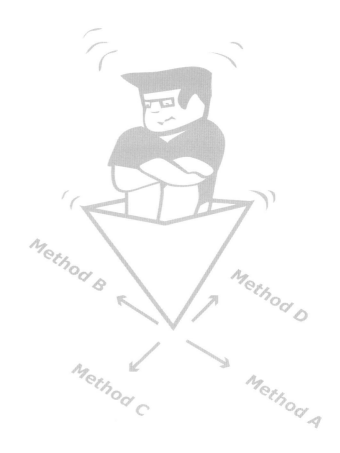

Meta-analyses are based on a statistical quantity known as an effect size, which is usually represented in the form of relative risk, odds ratio, or standardized mean difference. Relative risks and odds ratios are discussed in more detail in chapter 6: Analysis. A standardized mean difference is the difference between groups divided by a pooled standard deviation. Easily performed by standard software, calculation of the pooled standard deviation depends on study design and type of data. Relative risks, odds ratios, and standardized mean differences are unitless effect sizes that allow for transformation of many types of data and study designs, which then may be combined into a meta-analysis. A correction of the standardized mean difference and Hedges' g is often reported. Furthermore, they can be calculated from computed data, such as P values and confidence interval (CI).

Almost any outcome variable can be selected to calculate an effect size. The outcomes of interest may not be identical, such as pain VAS versus SF-36 bodily pain, but should be measuring the same domain, in this case pain. Therefore, one can pool studies that report outcomes using the Roland-Morris disability questionnaire and the Oswestry Disability Index, but not outcomes of pain VAS and Roland-Morris disability questionnaire. Moreover, the variable should be meaningful and acceptable by experts, computable from available published information, have good technical properties, and be independent of sample size.

In our vertebroplasty example, pain and function were continuous variables and reported with three different methods: baseline and follow-up for each group, improvement from baseline for each group, and difference in improvement between groups. Despite the different data types, a standardized mean difference can be calculated. New fractures were assessed as a dichotomous variable using the relative risk as the effect estimate.

9.5.6 Meta-analysis models

Fixed and random effects models are used to pool results in a meta-analysis (**Table 9.5-3**). The fixed effects model attempts to find a single common effect size that is invariant or fixed across all studies. This approach assumes that any inter-study deviation from the true effect is caused only by the variation within the individual studies. When pooling in fixed effects models, studies with greater precision are considered to be more substantial and offer a more reliable prediction of the true effect size.

Model	Assumptions	Weighting	Q statistic
Fixed effects	Study variation assumed to be related to within study error only	Inverse of study variance	Homogeneous
Random effects	Both within-study and between-study variance assumed	Inverse of combined within-study and between-study variance	Heterogeneous

Table 9.5-3   Characteristics of fixed and random effects models to pool data.

In order to incorporate this idea into the model, studies are weighted by the inverse of their variance. Essentially, the more precise an estimate, the more accurately it will describe the true effect. Therefore, it should be given more weight than a study possessing greater variation. In general, since variance is inversely related to the number of observations, the weight assigned is proportional to the sample size (**Fig 9.5-2**). Overall, as the sample size or number of studies increases to infinity the error converges to zero.

Often the assumptions behind the fixed effects model are not satisfied and a more involved approach is necessary. The random effects model assumes that there is not a common true effect among studies. Each study is, in fact, measuring something different. Despite all attempts to make studies uniform and consistent, differences will emerge, whether it is minor differences in methodology or variation across the samples tested. Thus, variation is considered both within the study and between studies.

In order to perform a meta-analysis in this framework, it is assumed that the results of individual studies are taken randomly from a distribution describing the possible pooled effects (usually assumed to be normal). In the random effects model, the center of this distribution is the combined effect measure of the meta-analysis. Like the fixed effects model, studies are weighted by the inverse of the variance. However, now the variance includes both the within-study and between-study variance. A common method to calculate variance in a random effects model is described by DerSimonian and Laird [1].

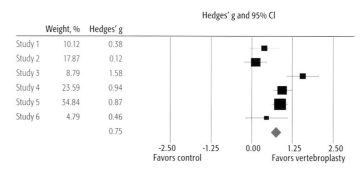

	Weight, %	Hedges' g
Study 1	10.12	0.38
Study 2	17.87	0.12
Study 3	8.79	1.58
Study 4	23.59	0.94
Study 5	34.84	0.87
Study 6	4.79	0.46
		0.75

Fig 9.5-2   A fixed effects model showing the results of six studies comparing vertebroplasty to nonoperative treatment. The studies are pooled based on the inverse of their variance, which is generally related to sample size. In this analysis, two large studies account for more than 55% of the effect, whereas two small studies for less than 10%. On the Forest plots, the box size is proportional to the weight used in the analysis.

Overall, the random effects model tends to equalize the weights between each study compared with the fixed effects model (**Fig 9.5-3**). Smaller studies become relatively more important because now they contribute to the distribution of possible effects and must be considered. The random effects model is more commonly used in practice.

A fixed effects model of the meta-analysis for our vertebroplasty example is show in **Fig 9.5-2**. The weighting used in meta-analysis is displayed in the table and shows that two studies account for more than 55% of the study, while two others account for less than 10%. In the random effects model, each study is shown to have similar weighting; thus increasing the importance of the smaller studies (**Fig 9.5-3**).

In primary studies we report the error using standard deviation, standard error, or variance. In meta-analyses we include both the variance between studies as well as within studies. Heterogeneity occurs when between-study variation is high. This is usually assessed using the Q or Cochrane statistic. A high value of Q relative to the number of studies indicates heterogeneity. Statistically, the null hypothesis that the studies are homogeneous and the Q statistic can be tested using the chi square distribution. Another reported statistic is I^2, which is the percentage of the observed variance that reflects real differences in effect size between studies. Values of I^2 equal to zero suggest that all the variability comes from the individual studies and not from between studies. Values of 25%, 50%, and 75% represent low, moderate, and high between-study variance, respectively.

Choosing which model to use should be done a priori, although it is commonly done based on the Q statistic. The choice, however, should be based on the perceived differences in study design, demographics, time points, treatment methods, protocol deviations, etc. In general, most cases of clinical trials should use the random effects model.

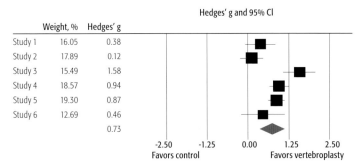

	Weight, %	Hedges' g
Study 1	16.05	0.38
Study 2	17.89	0.12
Study 3	15.49	1.58
Study 4	18.57	0.94
Study 5	19.30	0.87
Study 6	12.69	0.46
		0.73

Fig 9.5-3   A random effects model showing the results of the same six studies from our vertebroplasty example. With this method the weighting is more equally distributed as shown in the table and by the boxes on the plot.

9.5.7 Statistical analysis in meta-analysis

For our vertebroplasty example, the studies were evaluated for heterogeneity using the Q statistic (**Table 9.5-4**). The Q statistic (29.4) was large relative to the degrees of freedom (5), indicating a large amount of dispersion between studies. The test of the null hypothesis that the studies are homogeneous failed. The *P* value was too small (.0002). I^2 confirmed this as 83% of the variance was accounted for by between-study variation. This analysis confirmed the choice of using a random effects model in this example.

No. of studies	6
Q statistic	29.4
Degrees of freedom	5
P value of null hypothesis (studies are homogeneous)	.00002
I^2	83.0 %

Table 9.5-4   Tests for heterogeneity in the vertebroplasty example.

It is common to use meta-analysis to compare the effect across subgroups. Similar to the method used in a primary study, two subgroups can be compared using the Z distribution and a *t* test to examine significance. When more than two groups are present, then an analysis of variance or Q-test of homogeneity can be used. All these methods will give identical results.

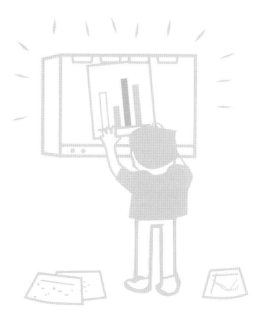

9.5.8 Reporting meta-analysis

Reports of meta-analyses should include:
- **Discussion of the effect size**
- **Analysis of the consistency of the effect**
- **Forest plots**
- **Publication bias**
- **Sensitivity analysis**

Effect size and consistency

If the true effect is robust and consistent among all studies, then the report should focus on the summary effect. When there is modest variation in effects across studies, then attention should be given to both the summary effect and its dispersion. Finally, when the effects are inconsistent, the summary effect may not be important and explanations for the dispersion should be examined.

Forest plots

Results of meta-analyses are commonly displayed using Forest plots. This is a graphical representation of each individual study and an overall summary result (**Fig 9.5-4**). In addition, tabular data can be attached. The standardized effect is plotted as a box, with the box size being proportional to the weight given to each study in the meta-analysis. How the weight is proportioned will depend on the model chosen. The horizontal error bars are the CI (usually designated at 95%). The vertical zero line indicates that the effect estimate is zero, whether this is a relative risk, odds ratio, or standardized mean difference. Any CI that touches this line is not statistically significant. The overall summary is a diamond with its length representing CI. Again, if it touches the zero line, then the overall results are not statistically significant. Other features may be added, such as weighting of each study. Forest plots are a graphical representation of the proportion of each study used in the analysis.

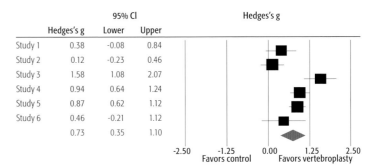

	Hedges's g	95% CI Lower	95% CI Upper
Study 1	0.38	-0.08	0.84
Study 2	0.12	-0.23	0.46
Study 3	1.58	1.08	2.07
Study 4	0.94	0.64	1.24
Study 5	0.87	0.62	1.12
Study 6	0.46	-0.21	1.12
	0.73	0.35	1.10

Fig 9.5-4 The Forest plot of early (3 months) pain relief comparing vertebroplasty and nonoperative treatment. The standardized differences (Hedges' g) ranged from 0.12 to 1.58, with a mean difference of 0.73. The 95% confidence interval (CI) of the mean effect (0.35–1.10) show statistical significance favoring vertebroplasty.

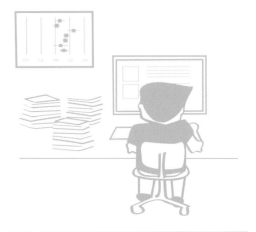

For our vertebroplasty example, the meta-analysis was performed using a random effects model because of differences in the inclusion and exclusion criteria, defined primary outcomes, time points, demographics, and treatment techniques.

The standardized mean difference for pain VAS was 0.73 with 95% CI (0.35–1.10), which was statistically significant. The standardized mean differences were pooled and the results displayed using the Forest plots. On the Forest plots, the summary result is a gray diamond located to the right of the zero vertical line, which indicates statistical significance. The Hedges' g effect from each study is presented in the table and represented graphically on the plot. All studies were in favor of vertebroplasty, with three studies being statistically significant.

The variation was large with wide CI. Box sizes were relatively uniform, an indication that each study was weighted about the same in the meta-analysis. The same result was present for function. These results indicate that vertebroplasty in early (less than 3 months) follow-up is associated with less pain than nonoperative treatment.

After examination the wide variance was attributed to the inclusion and exclusion criteria, which varied in time from fracture to randomization, diagnostic criteria to measure fracture age, number of treated levels, and differences in time point between studies. In addition, two negative studies used sham controls where patients were blinded to treatment. Similar findings were observed at late time points, although the effect size was smaller than early time points. The difference between early and late time points was statistically significant.

New fractures occurred in 18.6% and 19.2% of control and vertebroplasty patients, respectively. The mean relative risk was 1.06 (CI, 0.64–1.77) indicating no statistical difference in secondary fractures between vertebroplasty and nonoperative treatment (**Fig 9.5-5**).

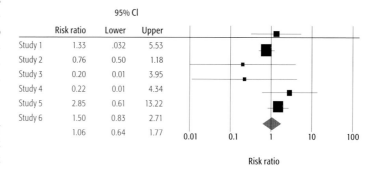

	Risk ratio	95% CI Lower	95% CI Upper
Study 1	1.33	.032	5.53
Study 2	0.76	0.50	1.18
Study 3	0.20	0.01	3.95
Study 4	0.22	0.01	4.34
Study 5	2.85	0.61	13.22
Study 6	1.50	0.83	2.71
	1.06	0.64	1.77

Fig 9.5-5 New fracture risk was assessed by relative risk. Three studies had higher and three studies had lower relative risk after vertebroplasty. None of which was significant. The standardized mean effect was 1.06 (CI, 0.64–1.77), which is also not significant.

Publication bias

Studies with large effects are more likely to be published than those with small or negative results. This results in publication bias, which will also result in bias of a meta-analysis. In order to characterize publication bias, both qualitative and quantitative methods have been developed. The funnel plot (inverted cone) displays the effect size on the x-axis and the standard error on the y-axis (**Fig 9.5-6**). The standard error reflects the precision of the study and is inversely related to sample size. The values are inverted so that larger studies (with larger sample sizes) are at the top. These have less dispersion from the actual effect, while smaller studies are at the bottom and have higher dispersion from the true effect. If all studies were available, then the distribution would be symmetrical around the true effect and distributed like an inverted cone. Areas on this plot with studies missing likely indicate publication bias.

Several quantitative methods can be used to assess publication bias. The fail-safe method imputes the number of studies required to nullify any significant effect. Similarly, the Orwins fail-safe N method determines the number of studies needed to nullify any desired effect, such as 0.10. If both of these methods result in large numbers of missing studies, then publication bias is unlikely. The trim and fill method computes the best estimate of the unbiased effect size by imputation of missing studies. If there is no shift of effect sizes with this model, then the original measured effect is valid.

Publication bias in the vertebroplasty example was assessed using the funnel plot (**Fig 9.5-6**). The studies appear to be distributed equally about the standard mean effect, indicating low likelihood of publication bias. Two outliers, one small and one with large effect are present. Quantitative methods also showed that publication bias was unlikely. The Orwins fail-safe N method showed that 39 studies with a zero effect size would be required to change the mean effect to 0.1. The trim and fill imputation of negative studies did not alter the effect size, indicating its robustness.

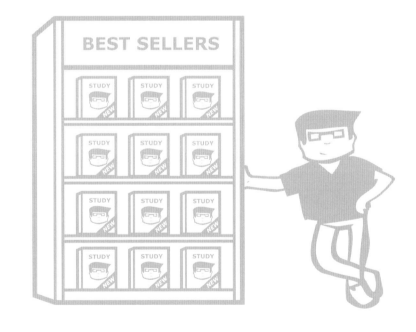

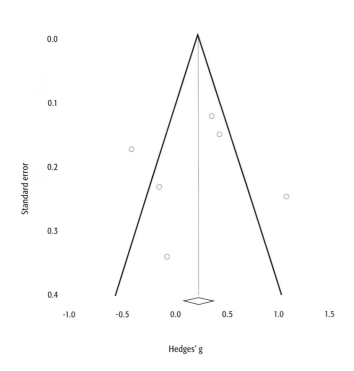

Fig 9.5-6   A funnel plot assessing publication bias for our vertebroplasty example. The standard error is located on the y-axis. The x-axis is the effect size. When all studies are available, the effects will be distributed symmetrically about the mean effect (vertical line) with larger studies (lower standard error) being at the top and smaller studies with less precision at the bottom. In the current example, the studies are symmetrically distributed, although two are outliers (one having a small effect and one a large effect). Sensitivity by single elimination of these studies did not change the statistical significance.

Sensitivity analysis

A meta-analysis should be evaluated for the robustness of the results and whether they are sensitive to the assumptions and decisions used in performing the meta-analysis. Examples of factors that can be examined are change in inclusion and exclusion criteria, exclusion of outliers, how missing data were addressed, and the statistical models used. Available software makes it easy to adjust many of the factors and detect the sensitivity of the effect sizes to changes in those factors.

For our vertebroplasty example, a sensitivity analysis was performed by single elimination of each study, which altered the effects size but did not change the level of significance. Further adjustments of assumed variables also did not change significance.

9.5.9 Summarizing results

☞ **When analyzing meta-analyses, the investigators should not only be concerned with the mean effect size and whether this is significant, but also with dispersion of the data. Inconsistent results (heterogeneity) may indicate that studies contain confounders that led to the variation between studies. Identification of these may be more important than measuring the actual effect size. Limitations should be discussed, particularly from the sensitivity and publication bias analyses.**

In summary, the meta-analysis of our vertebroplasty example demonstrated that vertebroplasty is effective at reducing pain 3 months following osteoporotic compression fracture. New fracture risk was no different between vertebroplasty and nonoperative treatment. There was heterogeneity between studies probably related to the differences in both nonoperative treatments (sham versus medical management) and operative groups (unilateral versus bilateral injection), inclusion and exclusion criteria, time points, and comorbidities.

9.5.10 Summary

- Meta-analysis is a powerful tool that can analyze similar studies to determine a direction and magnitude of effect.

- The currency of meta-analyses is the effect size, which can be calculated from multiple types of data.

- Pooling of studies is performed using fixed or random effect models depending on their heterogeneity. The fixed effect model weights the studies by the inverse of each study's variance. Weighting in random effect models is also done by inverse variance; however, in this case, it includes within- and between-study variance.

- Analyzing meta-analyses determines the direction and magnitude of effect as well as the dispersion or variance. If the effect is significant and consistent, the results should focus on effect size. When the results are inconsistent or have wide dispersion, then focus should be on identifying the causes of the variability.

- Publication bias should be assessed and a sensitivity analysis performed in a meta-analysis.

9.5.11 References

1. **DerSimonian R, Laird N** (1986) Meta-analysis in clinical trials. *Control Clin Trials;* 7(3): 177–188.

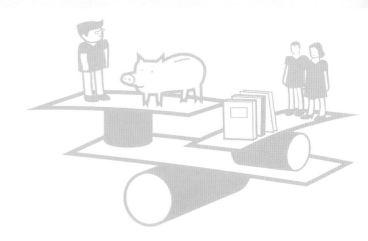

Healthcare policies need critical appraisal. Take an evidence-based approach to healthcare policy.

9.6   Healthcare policy:
evolution, evidence, and appraisal

9.6.1 Introduction

Healthcare policy is a complex topic that continues to evolve, particularly in light of shrinking resources for healthcare. Discussion of healthcare policy is appropriate for a clinical research book such as this for three interrelated reasons:

- Use of evidence generated by clinical research goes beyond publishing a paper.
- Implications point to the importance of enhancing the quality and credibility of reported evidence.
- There is an evolving need to apply critical appraisal skills to the review of healthcare policies.

Prior to the 1950s, healthcare decisions were based primarily on anecdotal information, pathophysiology, and the expert opinions of leaders in the profession. In the early 1990s, arguments for taking a more evidence-based approach to the practice of medicine emerged and the concept of evidence-based medicine (EBM) or evidence-based practice (EBP) began to take shape [1, 2]. Evidence-based practice is not intended to replace clinical experience and judgment, nor is it cookbook medicine [3, 4]. Rather, it is a "set of principles and methods intended to ensure that to the greatest extent possible, medical decisions, guidelines, and other types of policies are based on and consistent with good evidence of effectiveness and benefit" [3]. Evidence-based practice considers the validity of, and gaps in, research. It facilitates an informed interpretation of the literature within the context of the quality of evidence.

Evidence-based practice has the potential to enhance the overall quality of care by providing clinicians with the best current evidence to support decision making between the clinician and patient.

Consideration of a specific patient's presentation combined with the evidence and expertise needed to formulate a clinical judgment on treatment is the essence of EBP.

The application of an evidence-based approach to individual patient care has expanded to the use of evidence as the basis for broader healthcare policy, particularly in the last two decades [5]. A reasonable approach is to allocate limited healthcare resources to treatments and tests that are based on evidence from high-quality data that point to the safety and benefit to patients. Such policies in theory allow for provision of beneficial services while limiting the use of those that are not beneficial, possibly harmful, and not in the best interest of the patient.

Methods for developing evidence-based policy are still evolving and there are questions that need to be resolved:

- What constitutes judicious use of the highest-quality evidence available?
- How is the evidence discovered, selected, reviewed, appraised, and tied into the policy recommendations?
- How should clinicians and patients be involved?
- Should the development be transparent?
- Should there be criteria for critical appraisal of payer policies?

This special topic briefly provides some perspective on the future direction of healthcare policy and discusses the following with respect to such policy:

- Important definitions
- Role of evidence in healthcare policy
- Clinical impact
- Case example related to a specific spine surgery topic
- Rationale behind the critical appraisal of policies
- How critical appraisal of policies can lead to defining the next steps for clinicians, researchers, and policymakers

9.6.2 Definitions of health policy and healthcare policy

Both health policy and healthcare policy are broad terms with many definitions and interpretations. The World Health Organization states the following broad definition of health policy, primarily from a public health perspective on its website [6]:

"Health policy refers to decisions, plans, and actions that are undertaken to achieve specific health care goals within a society. An explicit health policy can achieve several things: it defines a vision for the future which in turn helps to establish targets and points of reference for the short and medium term. It outlines priorities and the expected roles of different groups; and it builds consensus and informs people."

Another source defines health policy as "a field of study and practice in which the priorities and values underlying health resource allocation are determined"[7].

On the other hand, the organization, delivery, and financing of health services are the domain of healthcare policy. Within this context, such policies may be developed and implemented by government agencies (eg, centers for Medicare and Medicaid services), healthcare insurers (eg, third-party payers), and healthcare delivery systems (eg, managed care organizations), each of which may have its own vision and agenda. The processes used for development of healthcare policies are as diverse as the bodies that develop them.

9.6.3 Role of evidence in healthcare policy

As described in chapter 9.4, systematic reviews (SRs), comparative effectiveness reviews, and health technology assessments (HTAs) provide a synthesis of evidence on a given clinical topic and inform EBP [5]. Well-done SRs, comparative effectiveness reviews, and HTAs are generally considered the highest quality of evidence in the evidence hierarchy. Thus, they are increasingly used to form the basis for clinical practice guidelines (CPGs), healthcare policy, and reimbursement policy. The implications of this for clinical practice have become increasingly apparent.

Few would contest that the judicious use of evidence to inform policy would potentially benefit the patient, clinician, and payer. There are, however, questions about how to do this. What types of evidence are important? What might constitute judicious use and how should it be tied into policy recommendations? Such questions pave the way for discussion of the critical appraisal of policies.

Given the description of healthcare policy, it stands to reason that the following elements should be included in a full healthcare policy:

- Highest-quality evidence on efficacy (from randomized controlled trials) and effectiveness (from methodologically rigorous observational studies)
- Evaluation of short-term and long-term safety
- Consideration of economic impact
- Consideration of subpopulations of patients in which there may be differential effectiveness or safety

In addition to these elements, consideration of patient preferences is evolving as a desirable component to include into policies.

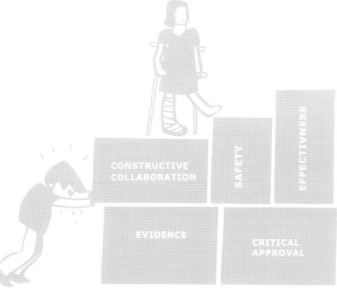
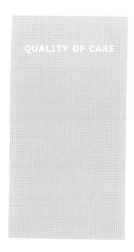

9.6.4 Clinical impact of healthcare policy

With an increased interest in the use of evidence for policy making, some believe that the art of medicine has given way to clinical quality initiatives based on peer-reviewed literature. The data extracted from literature are frequently the key in assessing the delivery of healthcare in hospitals and community settings [8, 9]. Systematic reviews of the literature on the management of specific clinical conditions are often considered the best clinical evidence for a treatment recommendation and formulation of guidelines [8,10].

☞ **Many in healthcare now advocate guidelines that ensure the provision of safe and appropriate medical care, and assess compliance with guidelines as a surrogate analysis of a physician's effectiveness in providing treatment [9].**

Within a third-party payer system, such as in the United States, a patient's access to medical treatment options is frequently determined by a payer's medical policy, rather than by recommendations from published guidelines or what the physician believes is the standard of care. Such policies are founded on the payer's assessment of the treatment recommendations as medically necessary [11,12]. Medical necessity for a treatment is defined as a medical service or procedure that is not for experimental or investigational purposes, and follows generally accepted standards of medical care in the community. However, payers have developed medical policies that supersede the local community's standards of medical care. Payers determine medical necessity based on their interpretation of the medical literature available, such as in the case of lumbar fusion [11,12]. As such, these medical policies act as treatment guidelines and arbiter to the physician in providing treatment options for their patient.

9.6.5 Payer policy: case example

Anecdotally, there is variation in the recommendations made in payer policies and in their quality. For example, the utilization of lumbar arthrodesis, or fusion, has risen fourfold in the past two decades and is associated with significant healthcare costs in the United States [13,14]. This comes at a time when healthcare costs in the United States have grown at a pace that threatens the stability of the nation's economy [15–17]. There has been debate whether this is due to the highly prevalent disease of lumbar spondylosis associated with low back pain or if the rapid growth of complex spine surgery (eg, anterior and posterior lumbar interbody fusions) and related economic factors are the cause [14]. This has led to the development of payer policies to temper the rise in healthcare utilization [18]. Physicians who specialize in spine care have found themselves challenged by these healthcare policies, which affects a patient's access to appropriate surgical care, defines nebulous aspects of what constitutes the standard of care for a patient, and defines the best available evidence to support it.

Based on a recent study by Cheng et al [19], selected payer policies each offered different recommendations for coverage of fusion as a treatment for chronic, nonradicular low back pain. They all cited evidence to support their individual policies. Why were their recommendations different? Were all policies consistent with how they found and used the evidence? How were they developed? This begs the question of whether there should be a critical appraisal system for healthcare policy. The authors believe this should be part of the future for healthcare policy evaluation.

9.6.6 Critical appraisal of payer policies: rationale, one approach, and case application

Critical appraisal of the literature is a necessary part of EBP and putting the results into the context of study quality. As described in chapter 9.4: Systematic reviews, there are guidelines for formulating and evaluating the quality of SRs. Clinical practice guidelines have also been subjected to critical appraisal. Clinical studies, SRs, and CPGs all influence patient care based on the EBM approach. Consideration of methodological rigor and transparency is part of this paradigm as well.

Given that medical payer policies significantly influence a patient's access to care, a critical appraisal of policies is also logical. However, there is currently no system for critical appraisal of healthcare policies. Cheng et al [19] explored the feasibility of creating and applying such a system as an initial step. The rationale for creating a critical appraisal system included the following:

- The primary goal of payer policies should be to promote the best possible patient outcomes based on diagnostic methods and treatments that work.
- All stakeholders potentially benefit when clinical recommendations are based on methodologically sound evaluation and synthesis of the best available evidence (ie, evidence with the least potential for bias to answer the clinical question), taking into consideration the potential benefits, costs, and harms of a given course of care.
- Although different organizations may have different purposes, resources, populations served, etc, the guidelines that they develop, the evidence base, its development and application to recommendations should be largely similar. (A caveat to this is that the publication date of a guideline may not coincide with the availability of the most recent evidence.)

- All stakeholders benefit when there is transparency in guideline development and policy making. Description of how recommendations are formulated and the potential for bias is important for transparency.

With that rationale in mind, Cheng et al [19] adapted the Appraisal of Guidelines Research and Evaluation (AGREE) instrument, which was developed and validated as an international tool to assess the development process and reporting of CPGs [20]. That instrument also contains components that would be important to the appraisal of medical policies. The criteria chosen focused on those that overlap with the Institute of Medicine (IOM) standards for clinical guidelines [21] and requirements for guideline inclusion in the National Guideline Clearinghouse [22], which related to the development and use of evidence for recommendations. This approach was considered reasonable because CPGs and payer policies are in theory based on the same body of evidence and there should be similarities in how evidence is obtained, assessed, and reported.

It is important to note that there is not necessarily a one-to-one relationship between the quality of a policy and the quality of the evidence used to support specific recommendations. A policy may be rigorously developed, well executed, and high quality despite poor quality of evidence. Likewise, a policy may be poorly developed, poorly executed, and be of poor quality despite using the highest-quality evidence. It is important to consider both the quality of development and the quality of evidence in assessing the overall value of a medical policy (or clinical guideline).

9.6.7 Recommendations for the future

For our case example, when the critical appraisal system was applied to selected payer policies on treatment of chronic, non-radicular low back pain, Cheng et al [19] found that payer policies varied substantially with respect to how evidence was sought, evaluated, reported, and tied into the specific recommendations, as well as the transparency with which they were developed. Some policies were explicit, well documented, and provided appropriate evidence to support their recommendations, while others were less so.

Findings by Cheng et al [19] suggest that there is merit in conducting a critical appraisal of payer policies in order to identify inconsistencies in their development with regard to methodology, use of evidence, and transparency. Future directions for clinicians and policymakers suggested by Cheng et al [19] are:

- Payer policies and treatment guidelines need to be transparently developed and based on the highest-quality evidence available.
- Clinicians, guideline developers, and policymakers should collaborate on this development. This process would also benefit from public and patient input.

While the AGREE instrument used in Cheng's study is a start toward a system for appraising policies, it has not been validated and insights gained from the process of applying it to policy suggest that further refinement is needed. In particular, some of the following factors are being considered for the next round of development of an appropriate tool for policies:

- Was the guideline or policy based on an SR?
- Was the highest level of evidence available in the literature cited?
- Were harms, costs, and patient preferences considered for fusion and for the alternative treatments recommended?
- What rationale was applied to the guideline recommendation or policy decision?
- Was there a logical interpretation of the available evidence?
- How should these findings be applied?

Evaluating the gaps in policies and CPGs provides important insight into what may be needed to enhance the evidence base available for clinical decision making, guideline development, and policy making.

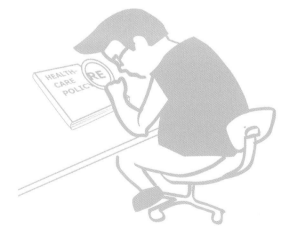

9.6.8 Summary

Analysis of the policies covering the use of fusion to treat chronic and nonradicular low back pain by Cheng et al [19] points to several areas where enhancing the evidence base may be important. One area relates to the identification of the patients that may benefit or be harmed most and least. Future studies should evaluate subgroups a priori to identify such patients. This may be accomplished through additional randomized controlled trials that are powered appropriately for subgroup analysis, registry evaluations, or high-quality observational studies.

Information about the types of outcomes and information that policymakers feel are important was also gleaned as part of the policy evaluation. Policymakers are beginning to focus more on what may constitute clinically important differences in outcomes between study groups, paying less attention to statistically significant differences. Thus, in designing future studies and creating clinical guidelines, the choice of outcomes measurements and determination of the minimal clinically important difference will be important.

Finally, evaluation of the guidelines led to the recommendation that the spine care community needs to develop or update high-quality treatment guidelines that adhere to the criteria described by the IOM and others. These are reflected in the critical appraisal tool that was used. New guidelines should attempt to be more comprehensive with respect to evidence on efficacy, effectiveness, harms, cost-effectiveness, and incorporation of patient preferences. They should be developed transparently following the rigorous processes described by the IOM and others.

- Healthcare policy development and implementation continues to evolve. It is safe to say that the use of evidence from clinical studies to inform healthcare policy is here to stay.

- The role of clinical researchers and informed clinicians in the creation and synthesis of high-quality evidence and in facilitating the formulation of responsible healthcare policy that is in the best interest of the patient cannot be underestimated.

- Creation of healthcare policy that allows patients to access the appropriate care will depend on the generation of high-quality evidence, use of transparent processes for SR, critical appraisal of the literature, linking of evidence on efficacy, effectiveness, safety and cost to policy recommendations, and constructive collaboration between clinicians and policymakers.

- Clinicians are responsible for conducting a critical appraisal of the literature and healthcare policies.

- It is likely that recommendations for further development of policies on fusion will be considered for the evaluation and treatment of other conditions as well.

9.6.9 References

1. **Eddy DM** (1990) Practice policies: where do they come from? *JAMA;* 263(9):1265–1272.
2. **Evidence-Based Medicine Working Group** (1992) Evidence-based medicine. *A new approach to teaching the practice of medicine. JAMA;* 268(17):2420–2425.
3. **Eddy DM** (2005) Evidence-based medicine: a unified approach. *Health Aff (Millwood);* 24(1):9–17.
4. **Sackett DL, Rosenberg WM, Gray JA, et al** (1996) Evidence based medicine: what it is and what it isn't. *BMJ;* 312(7023):71–72.
5. **Eddy D** (2009) Health technology assessment and evidence-based medicine: what are we talking about? *Value Health;* 12 Suppl 2:S6–7.
6. **World Health Organization (WHO)** (2011) Health topics: Health Policy. *Available at: www.who.int. Accessed September 27, 2012.*
7. **The Free Dictionary by Farlex** (2011) Heatlh policy definition. *Available at: www.medical-dictionary. thefreedictionary.com. Accessed September 27, 2012.*
8. **Guidelines for doctors in the New World** (1992) *Lancet;* 339(8803):1197–1198.
9. **Cheah TS** (1998) The impact of clinical guidelines and clinical pathways on medical practice: effectiveness and medico-legal aspects. *Ann Acad Med Singapore;* 27(4):533–539.
10. **Haines A, Feder G** (1992) Guidance on guidelines. *BMJ;* 305(6857):785–786.
11. **Aetna** (2010) Clinical Policy Bulletin: Laminectomy and Fusion. *Available at: www.aetna.com. Accessed September 27, 2012.*
12. **BlueCross BlueShield of North Carolina** (2011) Corporate Medical Policy: Lumbar Spine Fusion Surgery. *Available at: www.spine.org. Accessed September 27, 2012.*
13. **Dagenais S, Caro J, Haldeman S** (2008) A systematic review of low back pain cost of illness studies in the United States and internationally. *Spine J;* 8(1):8–20.
14. **Deyo RA, Gray DT, Kreuter W, et al** (2005) United States trends in lumbar fusion surgery for degenerative conditions. *Spine;* 30(12):1441–1445; discussion 1446–1447.
15. **Banthin JS, Cunningham P, Bernard DM** (2008) Financial burden of health care, 2001–2004. *Health Aff (Millwood);* 27(1):188–195.
16. **Kaiser Family Foundation** (2008) Health Care Costs and the 2008 Election. *Available at: www.kff.org. Accessed September 27, 2012.*
17. **Kaiser Family Foundation** (2009) Trends in Health Care Costs and Spending. *Available at: www.kff.org. Accessed September 27, 2012.*
18. **Eisner W** (2011) Milliman Made Me Do It. *Available at: www.ryortho.com. Accessed September 27, 2012.*
19. **Cheng JS, Lee MJ, Massicotte E, et al** (2011) Clinical guidelines and payer policies on fusion for the treatment of chronic low back pain. *Spine;* 36 Suppl 21:S144–163.
20. **AGREE Collaboration** (2003) Development and validation of an international appraisal instrument for assessing the quality of clinical practice guidelines: the AGREE project. *Qual Saf Health Care;* 12(1):18–23.
21. **Graham R, Mancher M, Wohlman DM, et al** (2011) *Clinical Practice Guidelines We Can Trust: Standards for Developing Trustworthy Clinical Practice Guidelines (CPGs).* Washington, DC; National Academies Press.
22. **Agency for Healthcare Research and Quality** (2011) National Guideline Clearinghouse. *Available at: www. guideline.gov. Accessed September 27, 2012.*

Glossary of terms and abbreviations

Glossary

....

Adjusted estimate   An estimate that reflects the degree of association between the exposure and outcome that remains after the effects of the confounder have been "removed" or "controlled for".

Allocation concealment   A method used to prevent participants, investigators, and others involved in the research study from learning about group assignments prior to the start of the study.

Analysis   Requires the consideration of everything from data quality, the description and characterization of the study population, to the analytical statistics performed and their correct interpretation.

Analytical statistics   These rely on the testing of statistical hypotheses (sometimes called testing of statistical significance) which is important when establishing whether a treatment is safe or superior, or when trying to establish whether a risk factor is associated with a specific outcome. Statistical tests aim to distinguish true differences and associations from chance.

Analytic studies   Studies that answer clinical questions and test hypotheses about how certain interventions effect patient outcome. Analytic studies can further be divided into two main categories: experiments and observational studies.

ANCOVA   Analysis of covariance allows you to compare one variable in two or more groups taking into account (or to correct for) variability of other variables, called covariates.

ANOVA   Analysis of variance allows you to determine if the means of several groups are all equal, and therefore generalizes the *t* test to more than two groups. Doing multiple two-sample *t* tests would result in an increased chance of committing a type I error. For this reason, ANOVAs are useful in comparing two, three, or more means.

Association   A relationship between two variables such that if one changes, the other changes in a predictable way. An association does not necessarily mean that one variable causes the other.

Attrition bias   A type of bias associated with the occurrence and management of loss to follow-up and deviations from protocol. Attrition bias leads to systematic differences in patients excluded from the study after they have been allocated to treatment groups, potentially changing the collective characteristics of the relevant groups.

Baseline factors   Those variables that should be accounted for in your study population and included in the first table of your manuscript. These variables are factors such as demographics, disease or diagnosis, comorbidities, concomitant medications, general health behaviors, psychosocial factors, physical function, disease severity classifications, and disease-specific measurements.

Bias   Any factor, recognized or not, that produces a systematic (but unexpected) variation in the findings of a study. Bias leads to an incorrect or distorted assessment of the association between an exposure and an effect in a target population.

Bivariate analysis   Such an analysis allows you to assess the distribution of individual variables and their impact on outcomes, which can lead to a more relevant and strategic development of a statistical model.

Blinding   A solution to minimizing various biases by masking which participant is receiving which treatment. Blinding can be undertaken at the level of the study subject, the clinician, the outcome measure (blinding of the individual undertaking the measurements), or the analysis (blinding of the person analyzing the data).

Boolean logic   The principle of Boolean logic lets you organize concepts together in sets. When searching computer databases these sets are controlled by using the Boolean operators OR, AND, and NOT.

Case-control study   A study that identifies groups based on their outcome and then determines which exposure (eg, treatment) they received.

Case report   A detailed report that describes an unexpected or unusual occurrence. This can include a unique therapeutic or treatment approach, an unexpected association between a disease and symptoms, an unanticipated adverse event, or an unusual combination of signs and symptoms. A case report can help identify new trends, alert others to look for similar occurrences, or provide a basis for a hypothesis that can be tested more formally.

Case series   A report of a group or series of patients with a defined disorder treated in a similar manner without a concurrent control group. Case series usually contain detailed demographic information on the patients and information on diagnosis, treatment, response to treatment, and follow-up.

Categorical data   Counts of the number of participants or observations in each category. These data are often described with percentages or other ratios (eg, rates). Common measurements in spine outcomes research include union and complication rates following surgery.

Chi-square test   A statistical method for testing the association between the row and column variables in a two-way table. The null hypothesis H0 assumes that there is no association between the variables, while the alternative hypothesis Ha claims that some association does exist. It is commonly used in bivariate analyses for categorical variables.

Clinical practice guidelines (CPG)   The Institute of Medicine (IOM) defines clinical practice guidelines as "systematically developed statements to assist practitioner and patient decisions about appropriate health care for specific clinical circumstances". The National Heart Lung and Blood Institute (NHLBI) website indicates that guidelines "help clinicians and patients make appropriate decisions about health care" and that they define "practices that

meet the needs of most patients in most circumstances". They may be developed by a range of groups (clinical specialty groups, government agencies, private organizations, policy makers, and even payers) each with their own perspective, goals, and intended uses.

Clinical significance   Relates to the magnitude of the observed effect that is clinically meaningful. A statistically significant result may or may not be clinically meaningful.

Cochrane Collaboration   An international, independent, nonprofit organization of over 28,000 contributors from more than 100 countries, dedicated to creating reports (including extensive systematic reviews) with up-to-date, accurate information about the effects of healthcare.

Cohort study   A study that compares outcomes over time between groups with different exposures. In therapeutic studies, these exposures are different treatments. The study design is similar to that of a randomized controlled trial except that allocation to treatment is not random. Cohort studies provide information on the effectiveness of a treatment in a more real world setting. Cohort studies can be either prospective or retrospective depending on when the study begins.

Comparative effectiveness research   The Institute of Medicine (IOM) defines it as the study of methods to "prevent, diagnose, treat, and monitor a clinical condition or to improve the delivery of care". There are two forms: direct generation of new clinical information via primary research and the synthesis of primary studies to allow conclusions across studies to be drawn. Reports synthesizing information across studies are referred to as comparative effectiveness reviews.

Comprehensive cohort design   Comprehensive cohort design is one where patients with strong preferences are offered their treatment of choice, while those without strong preferences are randomized in the conventional fashion. All patients (whether randomized or not) are followed up in the same way.

Confidence interval (CI)   An interval that shows the range within which the true treatment effect is likely to lie (subject to a number of assumptions). Confidence intervals are preferable to P values, as they tell us the range of possible effect sizes compatible with the data. They aid in the interpretation of clinical trial data by putting upper and lower bounds on the likely size of any true effect.

Confounding   Often referred to as a "mixing of effects", confounding occurs when the effects of an extraneous factor (confounder or confounding variable) blend in with the effects of the exposure of interest on a given outcome resulting in a falsification of the true relationship.

Continuous data   Data that, when graphed, form a distribution of values along a continuum. Distributions that form a bell-shaped curve are said to be approximately normally distributed, while all other distributions are non-normally distributed. Examples of continuous data in spine outcomes research include visual analogue pain scores and functional measures like the Oswestry Disability Index.

Cost-benefit analysis   An analysis that considers both costs and benefits in monetary terms.

Cost-effectiveness analysis   This term has specific meaning in health economics and is often misused in the medical literature to encompass any type of cost evaluation or economic analysis. Cost-effectiveness studies are a specific type of full economic evaluation that consider differences in costs and differences in effectiveness. However, effectiveness is measured variably between studies (eg, survival or a condition-specific outcome, such as symptom-free days).

Cost-minimization analysis   An analysis that considers the cost differences between alternatives of equal effectiveness. This assumes that two competing treatments are truly of equal effectiveness.

Cost-utility analysis   An analysis that considers differences in costs and outcomes for quality-adjusted survival, most often using the quality-adjusted life-year (QALY). Cost-utility studies have the advantage of providing an incremental cost effectiveness ratio (ICER) expressed as cost per QALY that eases comparison across multiple studies. They are usually considered the gold standard for economic evaluation, but are not common in spine treatment literature overall.

Cross-sectional study   A study that measures the exposure and outcome at the same time. Since exposure and outcome are measured at the same time, it is often unclear which came first.

Crude estimate   The association between the exposure and outcome ignoring (ie, not adjusting for) extraneous factors.

Data functionality   Represents the suitability of the data within your database. In other words, in order to evaluate your data, it has to be in a form that is suitable for statistical analysis.

Data quality   The three critical aspects to data quality are accuracy of the data, a plan for minimizing and handling missing data, and addressing and correcting nonsensical data.

Decision analysis   A systematic quantitative approach to making decisions when there is imperfect knowledge and uncertainty. It involves extensive statistical modeling of alternative strategies based on the probability of various outcomes at various stages of the decision-making process. The goal is to determine the most advantageous alternative under complex circumstances. It may be used as part of health economic modeling.

Descriptive studies   These studies describe a specific patient population without stating or testing a specific hypothesis. They include case reports and case series.

Detection bias   See measurement bias.

Disability-adjusted life-year (DALY)
A method for quantifying disease burden from morbidity and mortality. One lost year of "healthy life" is one DALY. Across a population, DALYs are calculated as the sum of years of life lost (YLL) due to premature mortality in the population and the years lost due to disability (YLD) for incident cases of the health condition. DALYs are used in cost-utility analyses to compare treatment alternatives.

Electronic database   An organized body of related information or data that can be accessed by computers. Electronic bibliographic databases contain references to published literature that can be readily searched to locate articles on a given topic.

Evidence-based medicine/practice   Integration of the best research evidence with clinical expertise and patient values and preferences to inform decision making between patients and clinicians.

Experiments   Studies that have some level of random chance used to allocate patients into different treatment groups.

Exposure   This can refer to a potential causal characteristic and a treatment, behavior, trait or, in the simplest sense, anything to which one may be exposed. An exposure is sometimes referred to in research as the independent variable since it is the factor being varied or manipulated in a study and which determines the change in the dependent variable (ie, outcomes).

Fischer exact test   A statistical significance test for categorical data, measuring the association between two variables in a 2x2 contingency table. Often used in lieu of a chi-square test when the sample sizes are small.

Forest plot   A graphical representation of each individual study in a meta-analysis and an overall summary result. The most common way to present the results of a meta-analysis.

Full economic evaluations   Studies assessing cost in the context of clinical outcomes. Cost-minimization, cost-benefit, cost-effectiveness, and cost-utility studies are considered full economic evaluations. They conventionally compare two well-defined clinical alternatives in the form of an incremental cost effectiveness ratio (ICER).

Gray literature   Written material that is not published commercially or controlled by commercial publishing entities, such as peer-reviewed journals. Examples of gray literature include academic, industry or government reports, policies, regulatory documents, professional association reports and guidelines, and technical government documents. Many health technology assessments are gray literature. Such information is generally not found via the usual channels of publication, distribution and bibliographic control, so additional search efforts are needed to identify them. It is considered an important source of information, however, because it may be the first and only source for some information and may be more up-to-date and easier to disseminate than information published via commercial publishing entities.

Health technology assessment (HTA)
A multifaceted and multidisciplinary process that systematically examines the efficacy, effectiveness, safety and cost, and other impacts of a health technology. The primary purpose is to inform policy making in healthcare. HTAs may address the direct and intended consequences of a given treatment, device, or diagnostic method in addition to consequences that are indirect and unintended. Evaluation of social, legal, and political impacts may be part of a HTA. The International Society for Pharmacoeconomics and Outcomes Research defines HTA as "a form of policy research that examines short- and long-term consequences of the application of a health-care technology."

Health-related quality of life (HRQoL)
A broad multidimensional concept that usually includes self-reported measures of physical and mental health.

Heterogeneity of treatment effect (HTE)
A variation in treatment outcome where some patients experience more or less benefit from a treatment than the averages reported in clinical trials.

Historical control group   A group that is chosen from a group of patients that were treated in the past and is used for comparison with subjects being treated currently.

Incremental cost effectiveness ratio (ICER)   Broadly defined as the comparative cost per unit of clinical improvement. The ICER is derived by dividing the differences in effectiveness by the difference in costs.

Institutional review board (IRB)   Also known as an independent ethics committee or ethical review board, it is a committee that has been formally designated to approve, monitor, and review biomedical and behavioral research involving humans.

Intention-to-treat analysis   An analysis of subjects in the group that they are initially randomized to. Intention-to-treat analyses are done to avoid the effects of crossover and drop-out, which may break the randomization to the treatment groups in a study. Intention-to-treat analysis provides information about the potential effects of treatment policy rather than on the potential effects of specific treatment.

Internal validity   The extent to which the results of a clinical research study are free from bias or more specifically, the degree to which one can infer that a cause and effect relationship exists between the exposure and outcomes.

Interquartile range (IQR)   A measure of statistical dispersion, being equal to the difference between the upper and lower quartiles. The interquartile range is a robust statistic and is often preferred to the total range when data is not normally distributed.

Measurement bias   A type of bias caused by systematic differences in outcome assessment or classification among groups being compared, ie, the accuracy of information collected about or from study participants is not equal between treatment and control groups.

Measurements   In the context of clinical research, measurements may include baseline factors, treatment factors, perioperative or immediate postoperative events, and outcomes, all of which should be defined and accounted for in a study protocol.

Medical subject headings (MeSH)   The US National Library of Medicine's controlled vocabulary thesaurus is used for indexing articles for MEDLINE. It is a set of terms naming descriptors in a hierarchical structure that enables users to search at various levels of specificity.

MEDLINE   The US National Library of Medicine's premier bibliographic database that contains over 19 million references and abstracts for journal articles in life sciences with a concentration on biomedicine. MEDLINE is the primary component of PubMed.

Meta-analysis   A statistical synthesis of related investigations that aims to determine if there is a significant effect and, if so, what is the magnitude of that effect. It assesses the variation within each study (heterogeneity) by measuring the consistency of results from study to study. The heterogeneity between studies may justify further investigation. Meta-analyses are best used to pool results of randomized controlled trials (RCTs).

Minimum clinically important difference (MCID)   Represents a threshold for a clinically meaningful improvement in a patient's reported health status or outcome. It has been defined as the smallest (absolute) difference in a score that is perceived by the patient to be beneficial and would result in a change in patient management in the absence of troublesome side-effects or great cost.

Multivariate analysis   A set of techniques for modeling and analyzing several variables, when the focus is on the relationship between a dependent variable and one or more independent variables. This analysis is typically performed using regression methods that allow for evaluation of multiple explanatory variables.

Narrative reviews   Summaries of selected literature that describe and discuss the current state of the science on a particular topic or theme from a contextual or theoretical perspective. They generally do not describe or follow a specified methodological approach for literature search and selection, summary, or analysis. They are generally not considered to be evidence based.

Observational studies   These are studies where no formal chance mechanism directs the assignment of patients to a specific treatment group. This can happen when the investigators assign patients to receive different treatments nonrandomly, or when the investigators simply observe the effect of a treatment that was administered without having control over treatment assignment.

P value   A statistical value that details how much evidence there is to reject the most common explanation for the data set. It can be considered to be the probability of obtaining a result at least as extreme as the one observed, given that the null hypothesis is true.

Patient-reported outcomes (PROs)   Questionnaires or instruments that patients complete by themselves or, when necessary, by others on the patient's behalf in order to obtain information in relation to functional ability, symptoms, health status, health-related quality of life, and results of specific treatment strategies.

Peer-reviewed literature   Articles submitted for publication that have gone through a rigorous process of evaluation involving a review and critique by other scholars in the same field as the author(s) of the manuscript (ie, the author's peers). These peer scholars offer their view of the overall quality of the article and its research. Currently, peer-reviewed literature is considered the highest form of scholarship.

Performance bias   A type of bias caused by a systematic difference in the delivery of care and/or the preferential provision of additional care (other than the treatment of interest) to patients in a clinical research study.

Perioperative or immediate posttreatment events   These are variables such as procedure time, blood loss, perioperative or immediate postoperative medications, and immediate postoperative complications.

Pharmacoeconomics   A scientific discipline that evaluates the clinical, economic, and humanistic aspects of pharmaceutical products, services, and programs, as well as other healthcare interventions. It uses a collection of descriptive and analytic techniques from multiple disciplines for evaluating pharmaceutical interventions in the healthcare system.

PICO   An acronym for patients, intervention, comparator (or comparison), and outcome. PICO is a framework for specifying study questions where treatments are compared or evaluations of diagnostic test validity are done. The intervention is usually the "new" treatment or test and the comparator is the usual, standard or reference treatment or test.

Power   A statistical property that refers to the ability of a study to statistically detect a true difference between study groups.

PPO   An acronym for patients, prognostic factor(s), and outcome. PPO is a framework for specifying study questions related to this evaluation of factors (ie, risk factors or prognostic factors) that may be associated with a specific outcome in a given patient population.

Prospective cohort study   A study that is initiated prior to the occurrence of outcomes. See cohort study.

Publication bias   Studies with large effects are more likely to be published than those with small or negative results. This results in publication bias, which will also result in bias of a meta-analysis. In order to characterize publication bias, both qualitative and quantitative methods are available.

PubMed   A free search engine maintained by the National Center for Biotechnology Information (NCBI) at the US National Library of Medicine. It comprises more than 22 million citations for biomedical literature from MEDLINE, life science journals, and online books. PubMed is one of the most widely used tools for searching the academic literature.

Quality-adjusted life-year (QALY)   A measure of disease burden and the value of health outcomes that takes into consideration both the quantity and quality of life lived. One QALY is a year of life adjusted for its quality of value. It is based on the number of years of life that would be added by the intervention and whether these years are spent in perfect health (assigned the value of 1.0), a reduced level of health (values less than 1), or death (value of 0). QALYs are used to represent benefits gained from medical procedures in terms of quality of life and survival for the patient. QALYs are used in cost-utility analyses to compare treatment alternatives.

Quasi-randomized controlled trial   A study where the assignment of participants is systematic but not truly random. Examples include assignment by rotation, date or year of birth, hospital or case record, and date of presentation or hospital admission.

Random allocation or assignment   A method of assigning participants in clinical trials into two or more groups randomly.

Randomized controlled trial (RCT)   An experiment in which a formal chance mechanism is used to assign patients to an intervention or control group.

Regression   A statistical technique for estimating the relationships among variables. It includes many techniques for modeling and analyzing several variables, when the focus is on the relationship between a dependent variable and one or more independent variables

Reliability   The ability to measure something the same way twice. Reliability is concerned with the consistency of an instrument or measurement. Reliability can be divided into reproducibility and internal consistency. Reproducibility can be further subdivided into interobserver and test-retest reproducibility.

Reporting bias   A type of bias that occurs when there are systematic differences between reported and unreported findings within a study, which are dependent on the nature and direction of the results.

Responsiveness   A measure of how well an instrument can detect changes as a result of an intervention. Responsiveness is also known as sensitivity to change.

Retrospective cohort study   A study that starts after the outcomes have already been collected. See cohort study.

Search engines   Programs or systems that search documents for specified keywords and return a list of the documents where the keywords were found.

Secular trend   Changes that occur over time related to healthcare delivery and advances and/or changes in surgical methods and equipment. These changes can be especially relevant when dealing with studies using historical control groups.

Selection bias   A type of bias caused by an error in the way participants are assigned to comparison groups (treatment or control) in a clinical research study resulting in systematic differences between the groups that influence prognosis or responsiveness to treatment.

Sensitivity analysis   A meta-analysis should be evaluated for the robustness of the results and whether they are sensitive to the assumptions and decisions used in performing the meta-analysis. Examples of factors that can be examined are change in inclusion and exclusion criteria, exclusion of outliers, how missing data were addressed, and the statistical models used.

Statistical interaction   Interaction occurs when the relation between one variable (eg, treatment) and the outcome is modified by the presence of another variable.

Statistical significance   Relates to how likely the observed effect is due to chance (ie, sampling variation).

Stratification   A method of "adjusting" the effect estimate during analysis. It involves looking at the association between the exposure and outcome for each factor category (or stratum) by calculating a stratum-specific estimate. This is one method used to assess and adjust for possible confounding in clinical studies.

Systematic review   A critical assessment and evaluation of all research studies that address a particular clinical issue. It is called "systematic" because the researchers use an organized method of searching for, assembling, and evaluating a body of literature on a particular topic using a set of pre-specified criteria. A systematic review typically includes a description of the finding of the collection of research studies.

t test   Assesses whether the means of two groups are statistically different from each other. This analysis is appropriate whenever you want to compare the means of two groups in normally distributed data.

Treatment factors   These variables will include the primary surgical procedures, additional procedures (eg, bone graft), devices used, and postoperative management strategies, such as nursing procedures (eg, compression stockings), medications, and rehabilitation procedures, depending on the study focus and other outcomes.

Two-stage randomized design   Participants are initially randomized into two groups. In the first group they are offered a choice of treatment while in the second group they are randomly assigned to a treatment.

Univariate analysis   The simplest form of statistical analysis. The analysis is carried out with the description of a single variable and its attributes. An example would be to summarize the mean age and distribution of the subjects in your data set.

Validity   Commonly defined as the extent to which an instrument or measurement measures what it is intended to measure.

Abbreviations

AGREE	Appraisal of Guidelines Research and Evaluation	ILIF	Interlaminar lumbar instrumented fusion	PLF	Posterior lateral instrumented fusion
AHRQ	Agency for Healthcare Research and Quality	INAHTA	International Network of Agencies for Health Technology Assessment	PPO	Patients, prognostic factors, and outcomes
ANCOVA	Analysis of covariance			PRO	Patient-reported outcomes
ANOVA	Analysis of variance	IOM	Institute of Medicine	PSI	Patient Satisfaction Index
ASP	Adjacent segment pathology	IQR	Interquartile range	QALY	Quality-adjusted life-years
CER	Comparative effectiveness reviews	IRB	Institutional review board	RCT	Randomized controlled trial
		ISPOR	International Society for Pharmacoeconomics and Outcomes Research	RR	Risk ratio
CI	Confidence interval			SD	Standard deviation
CPG	Clinical practice guidelines			SR	Systemic reviews
CRD	Center for Reviews and Dissemination	ITT	Intention-to-treat	VAS	Visual Analogue Scale
		LBOS	Low Back Pain Outcomes Score	WHO	World Health Organization
DALY	Disability-adjusted life-years	MCID	Minimal clinically important difference		
EBM	Evidence-based medicine				
EBP	Evidence-based practice	MeSH	Medical subject headings		
EED	Economic evaluation database	NCBI	National Center for Biotechnology Information		
EPC	Established evidence-based practice centers	NGC	National Guideline Clearinghouse		
EQ-5D	Euro-Quol 5D				
FDA	Food and Drug Administration	NICHSR	National Information Center on Health Services Research and Health Care Technology		
HRQoL	Health-related quality of life				
HTA	Health technology assessments				
HTE	Heterogeneity of treatment effect	NLM	National Library of Medicine		
		ODI	Oswestry Disability Index		
ICC	Interclass correlation coefficients	PCORI	Patient-centered Outcomes Research Institute		
ICER	Incremental cost effectiveness ratio	PICO	Patients, intervention, comparison, and outcomes		